GET *REAL!*

Unrealistic aspirations  possible standards _____-image, self-loathi_____ia and bulimia. W_____id to a chubby tee_____ weight, falling into_____ low self-esteem_____ bogus images of women in magazines or on TV.

It wasn't until I started to accept and love my body—and work with it rather than against it—that I got real results. I might not look it on TV, but I am a real flesh-and-blood woman with plenty of imperfections. I have learned to be the best me that I can be. I'm healthy and strong and in the best shape of my life because I accepted the reality of my body.

Forget perfect. Perfect is boring! Our bodies are beautiful, no matter how narrow our cultural definitions might be. Embrace your perceived imperfections—they make you unique—and love who you are. It's the only way to move forward.

"Fitness guru Michaels . . . brings her tough-love style to the pages of [*Winning By Losing*] . . . While no book has the power to change a person, the tips Michaels provides—create a support system, keep a journal, change your self-talk—do."
Publishers Weekly

WINNING BY LOSING

Drop the Weight,
Change Your Life

JILLIAN MICHAELS

HARPER

An Imprint of HarperCollins*Publishers*

This book was originally published in hardcover September 2005 and in trade paperback November 2007 by William Morrow and Harper Paperbacks, respectively, both Imprints of HarperCollins Publishers.

HARPER

An Imprint of HarperCollins*Publishers*
10 East 53rd Street
New York, New York 10022-5299

First Harper paperback printing: June 2010
First Harper trade paperback printing: November 2007
First William Morrow hardcover printing: September 2005

HarperCollins ® and Harper ® are registered trademarks of Harper-Collins Publishers.

Printed in the United States of America

Visit Harper paperbacks on the World Wide Web at
www.harpercollins.com

10 9 8 7 6 5 4 3 2 1

To my mother, Jo Ann McKarus, and my martial arts instructor, Robert David Margolin, two very special people who made me who I am, who taught me everything I know, who gave me everything they had to give and then some. Thank you. I only hope I can help one person in this life as much as you have both helped me.

Contents

Part 1: SELF
It's All About You

Part 2: SCIENCE
Dispelling Myths

Part 3: SWEAT
Why Exercise?

Acknowledgments

Thanks to my literary agent, Andrea Barzvi, and my agent, Jason Pinyan, for your support, guidance, and unflagging energy. Thanks to my amazing editor, Kathy Huck, and super-publicist, Shelby Meizlik, and everyone else at HarperCollins for your insight, expertise, and overtime; thanks to Claudia Herr, for putting it in the right words; thanks to Leeron and Lars, for giving me love, support, and opportunity; and, of course, thanks to ALL the members of the red team past and present. You are ROCK STARS. This wouldn't be possible without all your incredible dedication and hard work.

WINNING BY LOSING

Introduction
Committing to Change

Why have you picked up this book? I bet it's because you're looking for a change in your life. Well, you've come to the right place. No matter who you are, what you weigh, or how hopeless you might feel about your health, I'm here to tell you that you do have the power to regain control and change your life in ways you've never imagined possible. Here's the thing: deciding to change is easy; *acting* on it is another story.

If you are looking for the latest fad diet that promises quick and easy results, close this book and put it right back on the shelf. Don't waste your money. If you're looking for an easy way out, you're not ready for this book. Those books that promise you miracles are lying; you know the ones I'm talking about—"just eight minutes in the morning to the body of your dreams," or, "never count calories again." In our snap-your-fingers, instant gratification culture, that crap sounds great and sells. But it doesn't work. Think about it: If it did, and it were really that easy, we'd all be in perfect shape. America would not be facing an obesity crisis, and you wouldn't have picked up this book looking for yet another solution where all others have failed you.

Rest assured, I'm not going to lie to you. But by giving

you the truth, I may not be giving you what you want to hear. Changing your life for the better is not quick or easy—like anything that's worthwhile, positive transformation takes resolve, patience, and hard work. But as anyone who saw me coach my team to victory on NBC's *The Biggest Loser* will know, the results of my program are well worth the effort. The six people I coached on the show lost a collective total of 450 pounds in three months, and the winning loser lost 90 pounds on the show and went on to lose another 32 after he went home. These kind of results *are* possible. But you have to work for them.

Imagine, for a moment, your body as a car: if you're not eating right and you're not getting enough exercise, you are gaining weight and moving in reverse; if you're either eating right or getting exercise, you might be maintaining your weight, idling in neutral; when you put in a little time and effort and start eating right *and* getting the exercise you need, you will kick-start yourself into drive.

Now, step back and take a good look at your life today. And be honest. Are you happy with your status quo? If not, are you ready to let go of the quick-fix fantasy that has held you back in the past and really move toward change? Think about what you want out of life: whether it's to see your grandchildren take their first steps or to feel good about yourself so that you can be in a healthy relationship. Face your desires and your fears and embrace them. No matter what your goals are, you can reach them if you are willing to do the work, and are committed to becoming your best no matter how long it might take.

It's easy to make excuses. I hear them all the time, things like, "I don't have the money," or, "I don't have the time," or, "I'm genetically predisposed to obesity." Insert whatever totally lame excuse you like—*you* create your own reality, and if you believe you are destined to fail, chances are you will. However, if you believe you're worth it, you can achieve almost anything you want.

It's not going to be easy to change your life, but don't

worry—it's not going to be torture either. I make it simple and even fun. My program is designed for real people with real bodies and real lives. People like Ryan on my team on *The Biggest Loser*, who came up to me crying on the first day of the show, saying that he wanted to live long enough to have kids and go to their high school graduation. With my help, he lost 90 pounds in just three months. I've seen it work for my clients, and millions have seen it work for the people I coached to success on NBC's *The Biggest Loser*.

To put you in the driver's seat, I have devised the "3-S" approach, which is grounded in the three areas where you need to put in the work to get results: **self, science**, and **sweat**. And this is how the book is divided: The first section will outline some psychological and emotional aspects of losing weight and starting to live healthy. The second section will give you the tools you need to know the best foods for your unique body and your unique goals. In the third section, you will learn basic fundamentals of your muscular system and be provided with a detailed exercise guide that will enable you to custom design the fitness program that works best for *you*.

I know it's scary to confront yourself, look at your life up close, and really move toward change, but you don't have to go it alone. I'm here to guide you and help you uncover your potential for a better life and a better you. Once you start to see how strong you really are and what you are capable of, the sky's the limit.

I may not always tell you what you want to hear, but I will tell you the truth. The question you have to ask yourself: Am I ready to hear it? I can talk until I'm blue in the face, but until you're ready to pick up what I'm laying down, you're wasting your time.

Well, *are* you ready? Only turn the page if you're sure the answer is *yes*.

WINNING BY LOSING

part 1

SELF

It's All About You

There's already good news: you're still reading! Now let's get to work. Of the three all-important S's of my plan, Self is an especially important aspect to start with, and one that is overlooked by a lot of the popular health and fitness programs. Part of what makes my method unique is that before I talk about calories or ab crunches, I ground you in some methods for changing your thoughts and feelings about yourself and your body, so that you have a strong springboard from which to make the leap into a new and better life.

My own journey to health began when I was an overweight and unhappy teenager, so I know from firsthand experience the emotional baggage that being heavy brings with it. But with a little help and inspiration, I also found my way out of negativity and bad health, and not only am I now a better person for it, I also know the steps you can take *right now* to put you on the right mental and emotional path to a happier, healthier, more fulfilled life. Millions of viewers saw me push the members of my winning team on *The Biggest Loser* to confront and put their issues behind them. Those same millions watched my team shed 450 pounds in 3 months. Now it's your turn to get real and start losing.

1

Getting Real: Planning For Success

Your first step on the road to total health and your best life is simple: you can't achieve success if you are not moving toward something, so before you do anything else, you have to establish a long-term goal. Sounds easy, right? Not so fast. It's easy to say to yourself that you want to look like an action hero or a supermodel. It's a little bit different to arrive at an ultimate goal that is at once ambitious *and* attainable.

What exactly do I mean by attainable? In our day-to-day lives we are bombarded with images of supposed perfection and beauty all the time; it's easy to let the media and the world at large dictate how you feel you *should* look and consequently how you feel about how you *do* look. I'm telling you right now, that's got to stop. You know those articles about how to get J-Lo's toosh, Gwyneth's arms, Brad Pitt's rock-hard abs? Forget them! Even Cameron Diaz doesn't look like Cameron Diaz. Those photos we see in magazines are shot after hours of hair and makeup sessions, then airbrushed to perfection.

Unrealistic aspirations to live up to these impossible standards lead nowhere except to poor self-image, self-loathing, and disorders such as anorexia and bulimia. Lizzeth from my *Biggest Loser* season 1 team had suffered all her life. And I know because I've been there, too. When I went from being a chubby kid to a chubby teenager, I became obsessed with my weight, falling into a cyclical pattern of self-hatred and low self-esteem fueled by the bogus images of women in magazines or on TV. I struggled desperately, obsessively, with the desire to be as skinny as Kate Moss. In my worst years I starved myself and even went for a liposuction consultation. I would spend hours in front of the mirror picking myself apart, analyzing my every flaw, beating myself up over every imperfection; my body became a screen onto which I projected all my negative feelings.

It wasn't until I started to accept and love my body—and work with it rather than against it—that I got real results. I might not look it on TV, but I'm short and stocky. Period. I even have cellulite on my butt. I am a real flesh-and-blood woman with plenty of imperfections. And I happen to look and feel great—I have learned to be the best me that I can be. I'm healthy and strong and in the best shape of my life because I accepted the reality of my body. I will never have the petite, slender frame to which I aspired for so many years, but now I don't even want it. Once I let go of that unrealistic notion of what I thought I should look like and realized that I could be a sexy, voluptuous woman, I was able to look at myself honestly and see what could be done to make me look and feel my personal best.

Take a good hard look at where your negative feelings about yourself are coming from. Whatever the source may be, whether it's media brainwashing, judgment from family or friends, or maybe a bad relationship, you must recognize it so that you can begin to let it go. Forget perfect. Perfect is boring! Our bodies are beautiful, no matter how narrow our cultural definitions might be. Embrace your perceived imperfections—they make you unique—and love who you are. It's the only way to move forward.

So what is a realistic expectation of an ideal you? Below are three basic body types—identify the one that best applies to your body. It is important to understand your shape and what you can and can't expect from it.

1. **The apple shape.** The apple tends to store fat in his or her upper body, so if a person is carrying extra weight, it is usually around the belly. Fat stored in the upper body can lead to cardiac disease, so it is important for apples to be health conscious. Apples have evolved to store fat in this way to adapt to long periods of famine.
2. **The pear shape.** Pears hold the majority of their fat in the lower body: hips, buttocks, saddlebags. Pears are mostly women. This shape has evolved because fat stored in these areas aids in fertility and breast-feeding. This type of fat is not as much of a health risk as abdominal fat, but it is harder to lose.
3. **The proportionate shape.** Lucky proportionates have fat cells distributed equally throughout their entire body. When they gain weight, they gain it everywhere. When they lose weight, it comes off evenly.

As you can see, your basic shape is just a result of your particular pattern of fat deposits. With proper diet and exercise—the kind that I lay out and personalize for you in the "Science" and "Sweat" sections of this book—you can do a lot to alter your shape, but it's important that you get a grip on the fact that you can only win against genetics up to a certain point. Once you understand this, you can let go of unreachable goals and replace them with real ones.

After identifying your shape as one of the three basic types, you need to establish a realistic weight for your specific build. You've probably heard of the body mass index. The BMI is used to determine the amount of fat you have on your body according to your weight and height. Here's why you're not going to use it: it fails to distinguish between fat and muscle, so the BMI will ultimately give you an incomplete sense of your ideal weight. The medical industry has most recently set its weight guidelines according to the waist-to-hip ratio method, which is a much more accurate way of arriving at an ideal goal weight. Follow these steps to find yours.

1. Get a tape measure and measure your waist right at the belly button line.
2. Standing with feet hip-width apart, measure your hips at their widest point.
3. Now simply divide your waist measurement by your hip measurement. This is your waist-to-hip ratio.

The ideal waist-to-hip ratios are 0.80 for women and 0.95 for men. No matter what number you've arrived at, *do not be discouraged*. Beating yourself up is never a solution. As you lose weight and get fit, you will reduce and redistribute your fat, which will give you a lower waist-to-hip ratio.

I have outlined some reasonable target weight standards if you prefer to keep track of pounds. Keep in mind that depending on your frame and whether you are big or small boned, there is a leeway in either direction of about 10 pounds.

HEIGHT	WOMEN (weight in pounds)	MEN (weight in pounds)
4'10"	105	130
4'11"	110	135
5'	115	140
5'1"	120	145
5'2"	125	150
5'3"	130	155
5'4"	135	160
5'5"	140	165

HEIGHT	WOMEN (weight in pounds)	MEN (weight in pounds)
5'6"	145	170
5'7"	150	175
5'8"	155	180
5'9"	160	185
5'10"	165	190
5'11"	170	195
6'	175	200
6'1"	180	205
6'2"	185	210
6'3"	190	215
6'4"	195	220

GETTING IT IN WRITING

Now that you have an honest idea of what your shape can look like and what your goal weight should be, visualize it. Imagine in great detail how you will look and feel, the many ways in which your life will be different and, yes, better. This is where I suggest keeping a notebook. More than just a journal or a food log—that comes later—this is a place for you to write everything and see it in front of you so you are inspired to work through your issues and toward your goals, rather than avoid your problems and stay in neutral. Kelly from *The Biggest Loser* talked with me about wanting to go on a date when she went back home and finding the confidence to ask her boss for a raise. Since she's been home, she's done both those things and more.

Putting it all on paper will also help you think more fully about your goals: Do you want to be healthy, confident, physically and mentally strong? What clothes do you want to wear that you can't now? See and feel yourself in your ultimate body, living a new life, playing with your kids, going on a date, getting compliments from friends or coworkers. Whatever the ultimate goals are for you, both physically and emotionally, write them down now in as much *detail* as you can, and refer back to them often. They will help you stay motivated on your journey.

As you are envisioning the changes in your future, you must begin to let go of your past. Forget about what you looked like in high school, whether it was good or bad. Forget about fat periods or skinny periods in your life. The past does not define you; your present does. Having a vision of the future affects your behavior now. The key here is to let your daily actions be governed by your game plan for a new you and to keep that game plan in the forefront of your mind by writing about it and letting it become real. *There's no deadline.* Just commit to the process and take it day by day.

BREAKING DOWN YOUR GOALS

Attaining that long-term goal may seem overwhelming or too distant. There is a simple solution: now that you have a vision of where you ultimately want to be, you can start to set smaller short-term goals in order to stay on track. Plot your course of action by writing down the immediate-term things you need to do in order to attain your long-term goal. Be honest with yourself about the obstacles that will stand in your way, and you can begin to methodically eliminate them one by one. No immediate goal is too small as long as it helps you move toward your long-term vision.

As you are writing these short-term goals down, start thinking of little incentives to keep you going. For example, I don't love to work out. I know there are people out there who do. I'm just not one of them. Having said that, working out makes me feel great and inspires me in every area of my life, and I know myself well enough to realize that if I have a little external motivation, I can push myself through it. It is important that the incentives you come up with to motivate and reward yourself are not food related. Ryan from the show started saving his doughnut money to buy songs on iTunes at the end of every week. Start learning how to pamper and treat yourself in healthy life- and self-affirming ways that have nothing to do with food.

Here's an example of how you can break a long-term goal down into less overwhelming minigoals and the kinds of incentives you can create to help you stay the course.

GOAL	REWARD
ULTIMATE GOAL I want to lose 50 pounds. I want to feel healthy and strong. I want to fall in love. I want to wear a size 8 again.	ULTIMATE REWARD I will take a vacation to Hawaii where I can show off my new beach body and relax.
MONTHY GOALS I will lose 8 pounds this month. I will learn five healthy new recipes. I will lose an inch around my waist. I will be able to run a half-mile without stopping.	MONTHLY REWARDS I will buy myself the bathing suit that will fit me when I reach my ultimate goal. I will buy myself a Crock-Pot for cooking healthy at home. I will treat myself to a night on the town and go dancing. I will treat myself to a mini-iPod so I can listen to music at the gym.

GOAL	REWARD
WEEKLY GOALS I will work out three times this week. I will lose 2 pounds this week. I will not eat fast food this week.	WEEKLY REWARDS I will get a manicure and pedicure. I will treat myself to a movie on Sunday afternoon. I will take the money I've saved by not eating junk food and buy music for my workouts on iTunes.
DAILY GOALS I will rearrange my schedule to make time for the gym. I will talk to my spouse/partner about eating healthier at home. I will prepare healthy snacks to take to work.	DAILY REWARDS I will make time for myself and take a bubble bath. I will veg out in front of the TV and watch my favorite show uninterrupted. I will splurge a little and order in for dinner so that I don't have to cook.

These are only examples. Use the following grid to write down your long-term goals, then break them down into manageable, rewardable steps.

GOAL	REWARD
LONG-TERM GOALS	LONG-TERM REWARDS
MONTHLY GOALS	MONTHLY REWARDS
WEEKLY GOALS	WEEKLY REWARDS
DAILY GOALS	DAILY REWARDS

Meditate on your daily goals every morning to give purpose to your day. And every night before you go to sleep, think about your vision of the ultimate you—strong, healthy, and happy. Reaffirm your belief in yourself and your goals, and you will find yourself taking the active steps needed to achieve them.

2 | Recognizing Emotional Triggers

One of the most prevalent and insidious causes of weight gain is emotional eating. When I was my heaviest as a fifteen-year-old about 50 pounds heavier and 2 inches shorter than I am now, my parents were in the middle of one hell of an ugly divorce. I told everyone that I was fine, that I didn't care, but every day after school I would go up to the roof of our house and eat myself into a coma. I was masking my negative feelings and turning them inward against myself without even realizing it. It wasn't until someone who really loved me and reached out to me that I woke up, got wise, and set out on the road to healing. This person helped me find ways to look at my life and address my true feelings without anesthetizing myself with food.

INTERNAL CHECK-IN

We have all used food as a drug to help ourselves cope with stress at one time or another. You know what I'm talking about: cutbacks at work, a fight with your significant other, not having a significant other, problems with your kids— hundreds of situations can cause you to run to the fridge when you don't need to. I could get into the science of it all and explain how certain foods have the same chemical reactions in your brain as pleasure-inducing substances like alcohol or nicotine, but what's the point? If you are an emotional eater, you've probably figured that out. You've probably also figured out that unhealthy overeating leads not only to weight gain but can also lead to a destructive downward spiral of anxiety and self-loathing that is very hard to break on your own. That's why I'm here to help you.

There will never be a totally stress-free time in your life. The key is to identify the things that are making you feel pressured, sad, angry, or anxious. Once you have identified your emotional triggers, you can break the cycle and start getting back in control of when, why, and how you eat.

The best way to identify your own emotional triggers is through internal examination. Facing your issues by bringing them out of your subconscious and into your conscious reality is the most empowering thing you can do. This is another way to use your journal as a tool: write down not just what you eat every day but the emotional circumstances surrounding every meal and snack. From now on, every time you go to eat something, I want you to stop and ask yourself the following questions so that you can pinpoint the psychological and emotional conditions that are triggering your unhealthy eating habits. Write the answers down so you can't push them to the back of your mind when you're done.

1. ARE YOU HUNGRY?

Are there any physiological conditions you are experiencing that are signaling to you that you are hungry? Is your stomach growling? Do you feel weak or tired? Has it been longer than 3 or 4 hours since you last ate? It is not hard to determine whether you are genuinely physically hungry or whether you are eating for a different reason. If you've answered these questions and determined that you are hungry, then eat. If not, it's time for the next question.

2. ARE YOU DEPRESSED OR ANXIOUS?

Did you just get into a fight with someone? Are you anxious about a work-related deadline? Whatever it might be, write down in detail what you feel and why you think you are feeling it. If you don't get in touch with your emotions and their cause, you will continue to stumble along in life with an absolute guarantee of failure.

3. CAN YOU FIND A WAY TO ADDRESS WHATEVER EMOTIONS YOU MAY HAVE UNCOVERED IN AN APPROPRIATE WAY RATHER THAN SUPPRESSING THOSE EMOTIONS?

For example, if you had an argument with your mother, can you call her to talk it through? If you are feeling anxious about a work- or school-related deadline, can you get to work on the project to make yourself feel more on top of it? If you can rectify the issue in the moment by acting on it directly and positively, seize the opportunity to do so. Facing these kinds of problems is difficult, and it's always easier to try and numb yourself with food. But once you begin to look behind your behavior and analyze your feelings, it becomes easier and easier. Of course, it is possible and even likely that you will not have the means to resolve an issue or a situation at the exact moment that it is triggering you to behave self-destructively. If this is the case, go to the next question.

4. HOW CAN YOU TURN THIS PROBLEM INTO AN OPPORTUNITY?

Maybe you've recently been left by a long-term spouse or significant other. Maybe you've been fired from a job. Instead of seeing these kinds of scenarios as permanent blows to your self-esteem, try looking at them in a different light. Admit that you are in a lot of pain right now, but perhaps the relationship had been over for a while and there is someone better out there for you. Or tell yourself that losing your job does not change the fact that you are a smart, capable person who will have plenty of other offers in the future. Try and stay positive. Accept that sometimes you cannot see the forest for the trees, and you will be able to stay strong through the low moments. Try to find meaning and instruction in the pain. You will grow from it in amazing ways.

LEARNING HEALTHY BEHAVIOR PATTERNS

At the end of the day, sometimes life just sucks in ways that cannot be reasoned with or rationalized. The key is to learn how to take care of and pamper yourself in ways that are life-affirming, not self-destructive. You have to learn to deal with sabotaging emotions by establishing some healthy patterns of behavior and investing in your physical and emotional well-being.

Find some activities that comfort and interest you so that you will have the weapons to combat your sabotaging emotions without resorting to food. Think about what, apart from eating, soothes you. What makes you feel beautiful or sexy and desirable? If you steer yourself toward these positive feelings of self-worth, you will pick activities and behaviors that inherently contradict self-loathing and self-destructiveness. Take a bubble bath and listen to music you love. Go for a longer-than-usual walk with your dog. Go out dancing with friends. Get a massage or a manicure-pedicure. Learn to reward and nurture yourself with activities that make you feel good about being alive, and you will break the cycle of self-destruction caused by emotional overeating.

If you are a constant emotional grazer due to long-term boredom, loneliness, or depression, get a healthy hobby. Choose activities that soothe and comfort you—hobbies that offer you a means of self-expression. Do you like painting? Have you always wanted to try writing a mystery novel? Do you enjoy knitting? Is there a project you've been thinking about such as creating a family tree or fixing up an old car? You get the idea. Find some activities within your current situation that will give you a constructive outlet for your emotions.

We've now discussed some different methods for identifying, acknowledging, and bringing to the surface the emotions that have sabotaged you in the past. We've also discussed some methods for managing your feelings in a productive manner so that you can begin to change your outlook on life. We've even covered activities and hobbies that can help you change your self-destructive behavior patterns into healthy, life-affirming ones. I'm not saying it's going to be easy, but you can use this insight and self-knowledge to make real change for yourself. Once you force yourself to take some initial proactive steps, you will be amazed at how simple it can be to break out of the negativity and self-doubt that has you locked into believing that nothing will ever change for the better. You can reverse the cycle. The more you practice these simple techniques, the better you will feel.

3

Reconfiguring Your World and Developing Support Systems

We've all heard the phrase, "No man's an island." Well, no dieter is either. Losing weight is not easy, and we can use all the help we can get. Although personal transformation starts from within, our lives are deeply bound with friends, loved ones, and coworkers. Now that you have done some of the personal internal work required to get moving on the road to total fitness, it's time to widen the lens of investigation to include the people in your life who may be supporting—or sabotaging—you.

The desire to be accepted and loved is a primal human need that often drives us to conform to the behavior and attitudes of those around us. As a result, the people around you have a profound effect on the way you see the world and your place in it, as well as choices that you make every day. It is absolutely essential to recognize that you are not entirely alone as you set out to lose weight and get healthy.

Take me, for example. In high school I was part of the "wrong" crowd. I hung out with kids who were experimenting with drugs, getting into trouble, and failing out of school. Even though I knew a lot of what they did was not good for me, I copied their behaviors because I wanted them to accept me. For months at a time, my days consisted of skipping school, getting stoned, and gorging myself on the worst kinds of junk food. To this day I have trouble letting go of the troubled teen persona.

Fortunately, I found a situation to counterbalance and eventually outweigh the negative influences I had fallen under. At the suggestion of my mother, who was desperate to get me back on track and find a positive influence for me, I joined a karate class in an attempt to find an outlet for some of my anger and negative emotions. It was the teachers and students there who showed me the value of affirming influences and positive role models. Suddenly surrounded by such a nurturing and life-affirming group of people, I began to adopt their behaviors instead of those of my burned-out school friends. I began to take vitamins instead of drugs, I began to eat healthy and exercise instead of lazing around and eating junk food, and I began to study and do homework instead of skipping classes. You see, surrounding yourself with the wrong crowd can bring you down—way down. Surrounding yourself with the right crowd can inspire you to discover and nurture the best in yourself.

TROUBLESHOOTING YOUR CURRENT RELATIONSHIPS

Are the people in your life helping or hindering you? Let's take a good look at your current significant relationships and how they affect your life both on a day-to-day level and on a larger scale. Make a list in your journal of the names of all the influential people in your life. This could be family members, a significant other, friends, coworkers, anyone at all who is important to you. Here are some questions to help you identify problem people in your life and some ideas for how to deal with them so that nothing is forcing you off track.

1. DOES THIS PERSON PUSH FOOD ON YOU?

You know that friend who's always pushing you to have the fried noodles, or that aunt who always bakes your favorite peanut butter cookies, or your mother-in-law who makes you pasta with cream sauce every time you go to her house for dinner. Sure, it seems innocent enough. These people may not realize what they are doing, or they may think they are doing it out of love and acceptance of the way you are. The bottom line though is that their way of loving you is through food.

Solution

Lisa from my team on *The Biggest Loser* had this problem. Her mother was always pushing food on her, and I told her what I'm telling you: Acknowledge these behaviors. Recognize the problems and sit the person in question down and let them know that you are trying to lose weight and be healthy. Tell them how they can help and support you. Chances are they'll want to. Lisa's mother ended up learning new recipes so that she could cook for her daughter without sabotaging Lisa's health and happiness.

This is not always easy. Sometimes people will hear you and be able to change their behavior, but often their behavior has more to do with their own need for approval than with your need for support. No matter what their response, you need to be firm and hold your ground. At the end of the day, your health is your responsibility.

2. IS THIS PERSON AFRAID THAT IF YOU CHANGE YOU WILL OUTGROW OR LEAVE HIM?

I have so many clients whose significant others have been initially threatened when they take steps to get their health back on track. One client's girlfriend would always create a scene just when he was about to leave for the gym, so he was always late for his session. Another client's wife would refuse to buy healthy food at the grocery store or would constantly eat junk food in front of him. Is there anyone in your life who displays this kind of behavior? Is there someone who's always trying to persuade you to skip a workout or who always suggests pizza when it's his turn to cook? Is someone subtly sabotaging you on your journey to total health?

Solution

If someone on your list is sabotaging you in this way, ask yourself why. It doesn't mean he doesn't care about you. It could be that he is feeling insecure and threatened at the prospect of your transformation for the better. He might be worried that if you lose weight and get healthy, you will abandon him for someone "better." More likely than not, this person has no idea that he is undermining your resolve. Sit down with him, assure him that you love him, then tell him what's going on. Give examples of behavior he has exhibited that has sabotaged you in the past. Keep reassuring this person that you value him and he plays an important role in your life.

People commonly react defensively at first, but give them time. Continue to point out examples as they arise of the things they do that you feel impede your progress. If necessary, create boundaries within the relationship and stick to them. Do not let anything or anyone get in the way of your eating healthy, getting to the gym, or accomplishing what you want for the sake of your health and happiness.

It's easy to want to avoid this kind of confrontation, for fear of judgment, rejection, or abandonment, but you have to be brave and remember what's at stake. If you have tried everything and this person fails to respond, you might want to reconsider the relationship. Maybe this is someone who doesn't want what's best for you.

3. IS THIS PERSON OPENLY JEALOUS WHEN GOOD THINGS HAPPEN TO YOU?

I had a friend in high school who was always in competition with me. She would do things like tell me that I was looking too thin, then go buy me junk food, just because she wanted me to gain weight so that she would be skinnier. Do you have anyone in your life who always needs to be one step ahead of you and who would like to see you fail on your mission?

Solution

Take a good look at this relationship and assess whether this is someone you need in your life. Maybe this is an unhealthy relationship that does nothing for you but hold you back. If you want to and can get out of this relationship, do it. If it's a relationship you can't get out of, such as one with a coworker or family member, limit your contact with this person and set firm boundaries. Do not enter into conversations with her about your goals or your progress, whether good or bad. Do not give her ammunition to use against you.

Conversely, you may feel that despite her jealousy, the relationship is too important to you to let it go. If this is the case, try communicating the problem to this person, telling her how the dynamics of the relationship must change. Again, be specific. It's harder for people to deny their behavior when you can point out examples. No matter what, don't let her dissuade you from your path—you and you alone are in control of your life and your health.

BUILDING A NETWORK

Now that I've given you the troubleshooting tools you need to eliminate the obstacles that might lurk in your relationships, you can start to reconfigure your life around people who support you in your decision to get healthy.

It is important that the trusted people in your life know about your weight-loss regimen and your plan to get healthy. Sit down with them and clearly explain your goals and aspirations. Explain the weight-loss regimen you are following. Tell them what types of foods you are eating and what your workout schedule consists of. Make sure they are on the same page as you and that they understand your changing needs so that they can give you support.

But you need to give more than just an understanding of your diet and exercise schedule. It is important that you communicate the kinds of emotional support you need as well. I had a client whose wife would try to motivate him by nagging him constantly about his weight and poor diet. Instead of motivating him, his wife's comments only made him feel hopeless, which drove him to eat more. I asked this client how he wanted his wife to support him in his weight loss. He thought about it and said that he just wanted her to listen when he was frustrated with the diet or tired of the gym, and encourage him to stick with it without deprecating him. He wanted a partner in healthy living, not a nag.

The three of us sat down one day, and he explained all of this to her. My client and I then described how his wife could best be there for him to offer strength and encouragement. Sure, she was a little hurt at first, but it didn't take long for her to understand that her methods had been unhelpful and that she was totally capable of giving him the support he needed. By communicating to his wife in plain terms, this client eliminated a huge roadblock. The couple ended up happier and closer thanks to this honest expression of feelings. (He lost the weight—and so did his wife!)

We all have different triggers for positive and negative emotions when it comes to the people and relationships in our lives. If you patiently and consistently communicate what others can do to support you, you will build a network of strength that you can lean on when you feel discouraged or in need of reassurance.

Within this network there are three key relationships that you should foster or establish that will be of crucial assistance to you as you start to change your lifestyle.

1. A PARTNER IN CRIME

Is there someone in your life with whom you can go through the process of changing your life and getting healthy? Do you have a friend, coworker, or relative whose company you enjoy and whose goals are similar to yours? Misery loves company, but so does strength and resolve. Matt from the show roped his roommate into his fitness plan, and they helped each other eat right, work out, and stay motivated. The great thing about having a buddy is that you will be accountable to someone, whether it's someone waiting for you at the gym so that you can't flake or someone who stops you from reaching for a bag of chips in a moment of weakness. Having the right person or group to share your frustrations and progress with can be great motivation.

2. A ROLE MODEL

Another great motivation is having someone to look up to—someone who you trust to educate you about health and fitness, give you advice and answers when you're feeling lost, and stimulate your sense of possibility and potential.

My role model was a fellow student at the karate studio. Four years older than me, he was smart, funny, charismatic, and one hell of a fighter. He was testing for his black belt while I was wearing the blue. I took to him immediately, and he became my mentor, the big brother I'd always wanted but never had. I admired and looked up to him, aspiring to follow his example.

You could choose a personal trainer, a sponsor in a support group, or a trusted friend who has been there, done that—basically anyone who you respect, and who has the knowledge you need and the ability to challenge you and keep you moving toward your goal.

3. A FAN

The last important figure in this network (and somebody everyone needs, dieter or not) is a fan. Do you have someone in your life who just wants to see you happy and successful? Someone who encourages you and cheers you on no matter what? Look for someone who is always supportive of you without being asked. Maybe it's one of your kids, or your mom, or a best friend. Whoever it is, this person should nourish your heart. Love and kindness can bring you strength and courage when you need it most.

Now you understand that you do not have to go it alone. I've given you the basic tools and tactics you can use to change the relationships in your life so that they are geared toward maximizing your success. If you don't have enough people in your life who influence you positively or lend you support, seek them out. Join a group, hire a trainer, ask a friend from the office to be a diet buddy, or approach someone at the gym about training together. If you surround yourself with people who support you and want to see you succeed, chances are you will.

4 | The Right Attitude

Now that I've shown you the importance of support from others, it's back to you (what I lay down here always comes back to you). You can have all the external support in the world, but if you can't shake the negative attitude you have toward yourself and your body, you will never have long-term success in any weight-loss or fitness program.

So you're wondering, what is the right attitude and how can it help you lose weight? Having the right attitude is so important because thought is behavior—the power of mind is total, and the way you think of yourself manifests as your reality. We all know how easily negative thoughts about ourselves can lead to poor self-image, lack of confidence, hopelessness, and depression. You've heard about self-fulfilling prophecy, right? Well, if you tell yourself that you'll always be fat or that you'll never find happiness, chances are you will always be fat and you won't ever be happy. But imagine what could be possible if you harnessed your mental power with positive thoughts.

CHANGING YOUR SELF-TALK

A key element of changing your attitude is changing your self-talk—your internal monologue, the chattering conversation you have with yourself constantly all day long, whether you are aware of it or not. It's the voice in your head that says, "I'm genetically fat. Why not have another slice of cake?" or, "I can't exercise because I'm fat and lazy," or, "I'm worthless because I have no self-control and will always be this way." Blah blah blah. You know what I'm talking about—it's this kind of useless negativity that is holding you back, keeping you from being the best you that you can be. Now's the time to turn it around once and for all.

Imagine what would happen if you changed the dialogue so that it sounded more like this: "I can lose weight and be healthy. I will exercise to the best of my ability, and I will get stronger and better at it every time I do it. I am going to eat well today, and I will feel good about myself as a result." Your self-talk can make the difference between self-assurance and self-doubt, happiness and despair, success and failure. I can promise you that if you start making your self-talk more positive and affirming, and less defeatist and self-deprecating, your whole life will change for the better.

There is more to this idea than the way you talk to yourself. I also want you to think about the way you talk about yourself to others. We often adopt negative ways of identifying ourselves to others as a self-defense mechanism, a way of preempting ridicule and avoiding responsibility for our situation. Ryan Benson, who went on to win the individual weight-loss prize on *The Biggest Loser*, was a perfect example of this. When I first met him on the set, he was always referring to himself as "the funny fat guy." I put a stop to that crap immediately. I asked him why he felt the need to identify himself this way and how he felt it served him in his life. At first he tried to tell me that it was harmless, "just a bit of self-deprecating humor." In fact, these little thrown-off comments were damaging, and over time they had eroded all his self-confidence. Once he understood this, he became "the sexy funny guy who can do a handstand in my yoga class," and he ultimately lost 122 pounds. See what a difference the right attitude can make?

Now let's take a close look at the things you say to yourself on a daily basis, identify where you are being pointlessly, uselessly negative, and pinpoint where you can make improvements to achieve your goals. Don't get me wrong: I'm not about to tell you what you should think of yourself. I am simply going to teach you how to recognize and combat your negativity so that you can start to accentuate all the positive things. You are a diamond in the rough—we just need to clean off all the crud that has been hiding the gem. It's time to acknowledge your internalized negative opinions, your preconceived notions based on past failures, and *let them go*.

I have a few questions to ask you so that we can start exorcising these demons and move forward. I know, I know, more questions . . . but I need you to really get to know yourself, which can only happen if you do some serious investigation into what's going on in your head. Write your answers in your journal so that you can look back for a reality and motivation check down the road. You may well need a reminder in your own handwriting of why your goals matter and why you deserve to achieve them.

1. DO YOU HAVE A NEGATIVE SELF-IMAGE?

Do you constantly say things like, "I'm fat and ugly," or do you pick yourself apart and beat yourself up when you look in the mirror?

2. DO YOU LACK SELF-CONFIDENCE?

Do you doubt your ability to achieve your goals, weight related or otherwise? Do you dwell on your perceived limits or fears? Do you doubt your ability to accomplish the things you want to accomplish?

3. DO YOU FEEL POWERLESS?

Do you feel like you have no control over your life, or

do you make excuses like, "I'm genetically predisposed to being overweight"?

4. DO YOU LABEL YOURSELF IN NEGATIVE OR SELF-DEPRECATING WAYS?

Do you think and talk about your failure to lose weight as a foregone conclusion? Do you refer to yourself mockingly or otherwise as the happy/funny fat person? Is your e-mail address fatso@blank.com?

Now, look back at your responses. How would you describe the tone of your answers? Are they affirming and constructive, or are they downbeat and destructive? It can be hard to let go of these negative patterns of thought and behavior; often they are the result of years of self-loathing and internalizing the negative opinions and judgments of others. I don't care what kids called you in high school or even what someone mean may have said to you last week—that is no longer relevant. Release the past, focus on the present, and open yourself up to the possibilities that await you in the future.

This last question will help you understand why you have been propagating these destructive thoughts and behaviors so that we can cut them out at the root.

5. HOW IS THIS NEGATIVITY SERVING YOU?

Is what you say about yourself really the truth? What is its purpose? Is it a defense mechanism, and if so, against what? Are you just making complicated excuses? How does this kind of negativity help you achieve your goals?

All right, here's the last step: I want you to go back and reanswer these five questions—but this time positively. When I was in my early teens and just starting out in martial arts, I would beat myself up constantly over my perceived inadequacies. One day my instructor sat me down and made me write out my negative self-talk, then reverse it, like this:

NEGATIVE SELF-TALK STATEMENT

I am a terrible fighter. I have no coordination. I am fat and awkward, which makes me slow. I'm genetically not flexible. I will never be able to master these fighting techniques.

Reversal

I am a courageous fighter who is all heart. I am sturdy and steady, which gives me power and control. I have the drive and discipline to master any art form I desire, no matter how long it takes. I am a force to be reckoned with.

As soon as I was able to let go of the groundless negativity I had been holding on to with such attachment, my fighting improved in leaps and bounds. It is critical to your success that you acknowledge the harmful things you say to and about yourself, comprehend your reasons for saying them, and transform those negative thought patterns into constructive, helpful ones through reversal.

Positive self-talk is very simple—it's just talking to yourself in a confident, reassuring, friendly way. By reanswering my five questions in a positive way, you are effectively neutralizing your negativity and getting real so that you can move forward.

(BREAKING OUT OF) THE ALL-OR-NOTHING MENTALITY

Learning the art of positive self-talk will be instrumental to adopting the right attitude, but there is a little more to it—the right attitude also involves developing and maintaining a vigorously pragmatic frame of mind. One of the biggest hurdles you must overcome as you set out to change your life for the better is the all-or-nothing mentality.

Do you do things all the way or not at all? Do you start diets with superhuman resolve, saying things like, "I will give this diet 110 percent, I will go to the gym six times a week, and I will never eat pizza again," only to fall off the wagon and give up all hope? My team member Dave was one of these. He was either starving himself or bingeing and then feeling terrible about himself. Often we get to a place with our bodies where we have let things go to such an extent that we become disgusted and feel the need for immediate and drastic change to rectify the situation.

This kind of approach to anything, especially to your health and your body, can be very appealing, but I'm telling you right now it's the most dangerous way to set out. Human beings are imperfect. If you start out swearing to yourself that you will go to the gym six times a week and never eat pizza again, when you do skip a workout or give in to temptation—something *we all do*—you're likely to throw in the towel and start thinking of yourself as a worthless failure, which will get you exactly nowhere.

It is important to start learning how to make decisions about your health and your diet that you can realistically stick to and live with forever. Remember, you are not just going on a diet, you're establishing a pattern of health that will increase the quality of your life. I ended up challenging Dave to find a middle ground and showed him how to incorporate fun and the occasional surrender to temptation. He went away knowing that a healthy lifestyle does not have to be limited in any way, if you can practice a little pragmatic moderation. The right kind of thinking will help you not only attain your goals but will help keep you where you want to be once you get there.

Part of abandoning the all-or-nothing mentality is allowing yourself room for setbacks. We are bound to have lapses on the road to health and wellness, but it is critical that we learn how to handle small failures positively so that we can minimize their long-term destructive effects. One setback is one setback—it is not the end of the world, nor is it the end of your journey toward a better you.

Another critical step in renouncing the destructive all-or-nothing mindset is knowing how to walk a line between self-denial and self-indulgence. It is the middle ground between the two that offers the best foundation on which to build your new life. Denying yourself little pleasures such as an occasional glass of wine or a chocolate truffle will only make you feel deprived, frustrated, and ultimately hopeless about maintaining your discipline. A temptation is a lot less powerful if it isn't totally forbidden. This is where moderation comes in.

I will never be able to give up all the edible goodies life has to offer, but by practicing moderation I've found a solution to my weaknesses that I can live with every day. There is room for all foods, no matter how "bad" they are; it's just a matter of being conscious and careful of how often and how much. It's fine to have a piece of cake now and then, just not every day, and not the whole cake.

I can already hear what you're thinking: "If I eat a little bit, I'll want it all." My clients tell me the same thing all the time. We all have at least one food that we truly can't eat a little of without going overboard. Mine is ice cream. If you know that a particular food has a trigger effect on you, try choosing an alternative. I will often have a couple bites of cheesecake instead of ice cream so that my sweet tooth is satisfied, but I don't end up with an empty ice-cream carton in my hand. If your weakness is potato chips, try having some air-popped popcorn as a snack instead. Trust me—in time you can adapt so that small amounts of "bad" foods will not set you off on a binge.

The most important thing to remember from this chapter is not to waste time beating yourself up. There are no mistakes, just learning experiences. Weight loss is a process, and every process takes time. Sometimes it will be easy; sometimes it will be hard. You will encounter small failures—everyone does. Just remember, every pound you gain can be lost, and every slip-up you make is not a disaster. If you miss a workout, all is not forsaken! Get to the gym the next day and continue to focus on your short-term goals. Just because you made bad choices today doesn't mean you can't start over tomorrow. I know it sounds trite, but every day truly is a new beginning.

I've given you a lot to think about in this chapter. I know it can be scary to go out on a limb and believe in yourself. But faith in yourself and your worth is what will catalyze change in your life and keep you striving for the best. You might not be able to implement all of these attitude changes overnight, but be persistent. You will be surprised at how quickly you can change your mind and learn to coach yourself constantly toward ultimate success.

5

Behavior Modification: Techniques for Forming Healthy Habits

We've been over the psychological and emotional work you have to do in order to get on the right track. Now it's important that you know how to stay there. All it takes is a few simple changes to your everyday behavior and you can translate the internal work you're doing into lasting external results.

Lots of the so-called experts talk about willpower as being the key to losing weight. Forget it! Willpower doesn't exist—there's no such thing—at least not as a permanent unwavering personality trait. Sure we all have fleeting moments of bravado when we pass on the birthday cake and marvel at our own virtue. But we also know this particular virtue tends to come and go. What you're going to learn now are some basic techniques you can use to change your habits and program yourself against failure.

This is not going to be free: you're going to have to put in a little time and do the work—that's the deal. I'm telling you this right now because I don't want to hear at any point that you don't have the time. If that's your excuse, I want you to go back and read the Introduction where I talk about committing to change, then get back to me. I'll wait right here for you until you're ready, and I'll be here for however long it takes.

Ready? Okay, good. Let's move on.

Everything in the previous chapters has been leading up to this point. Like I said, it's not going to be easy at first, but as soon as you start seeing results, no matter how minor at first, you'll be amazed at the cycle of positivity and success you've created.

Let's gain some insight into the nitty-gritty specifics of your current self-defeating behaviors that have been your downfall in the past. By doing this, we can substitute healthy, affirming behaviors instead. Listed below are several of the most common causes of overeating. I want you to write down in your journal however many of the excuses apply or have applied to you. That way we can isolate your specific problems and work on finding solutions for all of them.

1. EMOTION
Do you overeat as a coping mechanism, to numb suffering, allay fears, combat loneliness, and so on?

2. REWARD
Do you eat to make you feel good about yourself whenever you've done a good job on something?

3. SEEKING ACCEPTANCE
Do you overeat because you're seeking social acceptance? Do you eat fattening foods at parties in order not to offend the host? If you're out with friends, do you feel the need to have a drink just to fit in?

4. EXTERNAL CUES
Are you stimulated to eat by things like fast-food com-

mercials as opposed to hunger signals from your own body?

5. MINDLESSNESS

Do you go through the day grazing constantly on anything that's around and lose track of how many calories you're consuming?

6. BOREDOM

Do you eat because you can't find anything else to do?

7. ARE THERE REASONS I MAY NOT HAVE LISTED THAT APPLY TO YOUR PARTICULAR PROBLEMS WITH OVEREATING? IF THERE ARE, WRITE THEM DOWN.

Whatever your downfalls might have been in the past, there is a way to deal with them in the present. Now that you know the things that tend to sabotage you, read this chapter carefully to find the solutions that apply to your specific set of circumstances.

AVOIDING DANGEROUS SITUATIONS

Eliminate as many obstacles as you can before they get in your way. Think of yourself as being on a mission—the key to success is having a game plan for every situation that might throw you off course. Many of our problems have simple solutions we can't see because we're wrapped up in them. Ryan is a great example. His daily drive to work took him past a doughnut shop, and sure enough he would find himself stopping there almost every day. When we got to work on the show, I ordered him to take another route to work so that he wasn't putting temptation in his path. The result? He lost 2 pounds in one week just from that simple change to his daily routine.

I had another client who would skip breakfast regularly because she claimed she didn't have time in the morning.

When lunch rolled around, she would be ravenous and wind up eating everything in sight, overwhelming a metabolism that was sluggish from not having been revved up by a morning meal. My solution? I took her grocery shopping and showed her the healthy low-calorie foods she could run out the door with every morning, like an apple, a low-fat yogurt, or a single serving of low-cal cottage cheese.

This stuff isn't brain surgery—it's common sense. If you take the time to think ahead, you can come up with ways to combat every potentially sabotaging situation. Here are some examples.

1. Go through your kitchen and throw out all the junk food and processed garbage immediately—you can't eat it if it's not there. Don't buy these foods anymore at the store—just eliminate them from your kitchen entirely. Even if you have to put up with a little whining from the kids or your spouse or whoever, they're better off not eating that crap as well. Reacquaint yourself with your local supermarket, find the healthy sections, and try to avoid the snack food aisles or whatever foods make you feel powerless.

2. If you get into trouble during the day at the office, see if you can really make an effort to avoid the high-voltage areas. If there is a vending machine in the office kitchen that gets you every time or if the cafeteria offers a lot of fattening foods, stay away from these places. Bring healthy snacks and meals of your own to keep at your desk. Do whatever you can to steer clear of anything that might throw you off course and hamper your success.

3. If you are tempted by fast-food joints or other unwholesome foods on your daily commute to and from work, find yourself a different route if you can, even if it adds a few minutes to your journey. You can't stop for a cheeseburger if you don't go by the fast-food chain. It's worth a longer commute to have this temptation out of your face.

4. When you go to restaurants, ask the waiter not to bring chips, bread, or anything else you don't want to graze on just because it's there.
5. When you're on the road or away from home for any reason, pack healthy snacks to take with you so that you're not relying on whatever's available when hunger strikes. Whether you're flying or going to the mall, bring something healthy with you so that you don't have to eat junk if it's all that's around.
6. If food commercials on television make you hungry and drive you to snack uncontrollably, videorecord your shows so that you can skip the commercials, or keep a few magazines close by so that you have something to zone out with until the commercials are over.

LEARNING BEHAVIORS THAT ARE INCOMPATIBLE WITH OVEREATING

Start coming up with some of your own healthy behaviors. This is particularly useful if your problem relates to emotional eating. Whether it's out of boredom, anxiety, depression, anger, or even pleasure, you can learn to employ activities that are incompatible with overeating or being otherwise self-destructive. Here are some examples.

1. **Get active.** Start incorporating more physical exercise into your daily routine. Get a hobby that combines being physically active with socializing. Start taking your dog for longer walks. Get an exercise bike or join a dance class. I could go on and on. There are any number of ways you can get your body going, but find activities you like so that you will have less trouble being motivated to move. Physical exercise helps reduce stress and keeps you feeling balanced so that you will be less prone to emotional overeating.
2. **Relax and pamper yourself.** Take a long bubble bath; treat yourself to a manicure or a massage; buy yourself a

little something you've been wanting; give yourself time to read a book. Find ways to treat yourself like a king or a queen without resorting to food.

3. **Be productive and responsible.** Find something in your life that you've been meaning to do—a big project or a nagging chore—and stop letting its undoneness make you feel bad or lazy. Fix up your house, pay your bills, clean out the attic, go through your closets and take a bag of stuff you don't want to the Salvation Army, or just do laundry. If you start to take charge of the external things in your life, it will be easier to take charge of the internal ones.

You'll notice that these suggestions will pay off in terms of weight loss, but they will also lead to your becoming a more relaxed, healthier, and happier human being. By taking the time to look after yourself, you are reminding yourself and stating to the world that you are worth it, that you know you deserve the best life has to offer. Once you project this kind of attitude, you'll see that your reality will adapt to affirm you.

CURBING MINDLESS EATING

Here's another thing: the grazing has got to stop. Having a scheduled snack is one thing, but picking at things throughout the day just because they're around can add up to major calories before you know it. If this is your problem, try some of the following tactics, see which ones work for you, or let them guide you to your own solutions.

To curb daytime grazing:

1. Don't eat while standing up, in the car, or when you're on the go or you don't have time to have a proper meal. If you're more relaxed while you eat, you will be less likely to throw whatever food is at hand into your mouth in-between meals.

2. Don't skip meals! You might think you're saving yourself calories, but you'll wind up so hungry that you'll probably consume extra calories to feel full.

To curb nighttime grazing:

3. Nighttime grazing is often a result of boredom. Perhaps now is a good time to take up that hobby you've been thinking about.
4. Brush your teeth. Food never seems quite as appealing when you have toothpaste mouth.
5. Try making yourself a cup of hot tea; the warm liquid in your stomach can help you feel satiated.

To curb grazing at parties and social events:

6. Take a fiber supplement or have a healthy snack before you go so that right off the bat you're not hungry and tempted.
7. Focus on the company, not the food.
8. Hang out as far away from the food as you can, preferably in a separate room.
9. If it's appropriate, bring your own healthy dish to share with the party.

LEARNING TO SLOW DOWN

Eating too quickly is one of the leading causes of overeating. It takes twenty minutes for your stomach to register the food you eat and send the "I'm full" message to your brain. If you are barreling through your meals in fifteen minutes, you are probably eating way more than is necessary to satisfy your hunger. Force yourself to slow down. Savor and enjoy your meal. Here are some tricks to keep in mind.

1. If you're right-handed, eat with your left hand, and vice versa.

2. Cut your food into small pieces, and eat your meal one morsel at a time.
3. Make yourself put your silverware down in between bites.
4. Take a sip of a beverage in between bites. Water is always best.

I know these hints may sound silly, but they work. Slow yourself down and you will find that you feel satisfied before you are tempted to reach for a second helping.

CUTTING PORTION SIZE

Americans have totally skewed ideas about portion size. I have never been to a country that has portions as enormous as we do. Honestly, go anywhere else in the world and check this out. We are a gluttonous society conditioned to think that more equals better. Just look at the "super-size me" phenomenon—the insidious up-selling of fast food in chain restaurants, movie theaters, and countless other consumer-driven environments. Customers are encouraged to eat more in order to take advantage of a "bargain." The idea that you need 100 french fries in one sitting just to save a quarter you wouldn't have spent in the first place is a mistaken notion that Americans are paying for with their health and sometimes their lives. Here are a few techniques you can put into play to safeguard against overeating due to lack of portion control.

1. If you're at home, use smaller plates to create the illusion of a bigger serving.
2. If you're at a restaurant and you know the portions are huge, ask the server to put half of your meal in a doggy bag before it's even brought to you. This saves you money as well as unnecessary calorie overload.
3. Try sharing an entrée with your dining partner.
4. Make a new rule for yourself that there always has to be

something left on your plate. Leaving something on your plate will bring it home that you are in control of the food, not the other way around. A little bit of empowerment can go a long way!

At the end of the day, these tips are nothing more than common-sense wisdom that I've gathered over the years as I've strived to maintain the best health and well-being possible. I know that some of the suggestions may sound thought- or time-consuming and generally inconvenient. But aren't we here together in the first place because you want to look and feel great about yourself? Be conscientious and keep your eye on the prize. Remember that you're totally worth it.

If you listen to one thing and one thing only (but you'd better be listening to more than that!), listen to this: Choose the healthy option. Go for low-cal, low-fat foods instead of junk. Junk is usually more readily available, so this will take persistence—but what worthwhile mission doesn't? If you're going to graze, have half an apple instead of a candy bar. Have a bowl of air-popped popcorn instead of a bag of potato chips. Have a sugar-free dessert instead of ice cream. If you're going to drink soda, make it diet. In the next part, we'll get specific about nutrition and what you should and shouldn't be eating. Old habits die hard, but keep at it. When your patience and hard work start to pay off, the results will affirm you in ways you never imagined possible.

part 2

SCIENCE

Dispelling Myths

In the last section, we went over the internal work you need to do in order to really effect change in your life, and while it's true that getting healthy has a lot to do with where your head is at, there is more to it. Now it's time to talk about the next "S" you have to focus on: the science behind our bodies so you have the knowledge to transform your body and regain control over your life.

First, it is crucial for you to understand that there is no product, procedure, or miracle-diet that is going to do the work for you to lose weight—you cannot cheat and expect to win. On my own personal journey toward weight loss, I must have tried over twenty different diets, taken every so-called "fat-burning" and "metabolism-enhancing" pill on the market, and experimented with every exercise gadget ever sold. I even flirted with the idea of liposuction. To figure out what really works, I went damn-near crazy trying to decipher all the conflicting information and half-baked nutritional theories. I'm sure at some point you've experienced the same confusion. So before we kick start your new lifestyle, let's cut through the bull once and for all by dispelling some of the diet myths and misconceptions that may be holding you back.

THE STARVATION TRAP

The first myth on the chopping block is the idea that starvation is the fastest way to lose weight. I can't tell you how many of my clients have attempted to starve themselves thin; they go on crazy crash diets that severely restrict caloric intake, or experiment with liquid diets and fasting. What they don't know is that this is a one-way ticket to failure: Not eating enough triggers your body's starvation survival mechanism, causing your metabolism to slow down to hoard fat and keep your vital organs protected and insulated. Because your body is holding on to all the fat it can, it begins to draw energy from your muscles instead; you will lose weight, but it will be valuable muscle tissue. Muscles are your body's metabolic furnace—they burn calories even when you're sleeping—and the less muscle you have, the slower your metabolism will be. As soon as you go off the starvation diet, which you must at some point, you will gain back all the weight you lost, and usually more, because you have made your body less efficient at using energy. This insane process of losing weight only to gain it right back is called yo-yo dieting; it can make you feel weak and tired, can severely jeopardize your immune system, and can leave you feeling frustrated and despondent about ever losing the weight for good.

MAGIC PILLS AND MIRACLE SURGERIES

Diet pills and surgical weight-loss options are two more examples of detrimental quick fixes. Diet products and procedures are for the most part simply gimmicks that target people's apathy and hopelessness about their own health. All you have to do is look at the fine print on the packaging of most of these products to see that they are completely bogus. Take a look next time you're at the store: you'll find there is almost always a disclaimer that says something like, "This product can successfully help you lose weight when accompanied by a sensible diet and exercise program." The product itself has nothing to do with your weight-loss success. There are some supplements on the market that can help maximize your weight-loss regimen, but if you are not eating right and exercising, they are totally ineffective.

If you think that surgery is a safe way of shedding pounds without having to do any work, think again. One in fifty patients who undergo gastric bypass surgery will die within a month of the operation, and even patients who make a full recovery are left struggling unaided with the issues that caused them to be overweight in the first place, because psychologically and emotionally these quick-fix measures target only the symptom, not the root cause of weight problems—that's why my program begins with the internal work and why you're going to see the results you haven't seen in the past.

Many of my clients come to me having tried everything and are desperate to know how to cut through all the crap and figure out what works. Kelly Minner from my team on *The Biggest Loser* burst into tears telling me about all the diets and products she tried in the past . . . but this was before she lost 85 pounds in 5 months. What I told Kelly and what I'm telling you is that once you let go of the easy-way-out fantasy and start working with your body not against it, nothing can stand in the way of your success.

Obviously you can't start working with your body unless you have a basic understanding of how it functions. In the following chapters I will lead you on a crash course in the science of weight loss. That's right, I said *science*. But don't worry—we're talking basic stuff here, and I will make it easy to follow.

Our main focus will be on you as an individual with a unique biology and your own distinct nutritional needs.

I will tell you everything you need to know about how to whip your metabolism into shape and get it on your side and working for you. I will also break down the various diets that are out there so that you can see which elements from which type of diet works best for you. This is a critical step on the road to lasting health, so do yourself a favor and bear with me here.

Your life and your happiness are things you have to be willing to put some time into and do a little work for. Believe me, the payoff is more than worth it. Once you have a firm grasp on the basic facts, you will have the tools you need to negotiate your way through the myths and misrepresentations that may have tripped you up in the past as well as the knowledge to custom-design your own diet and fitness regimen so that you are in control and can achieve your maximum success.

6

Weight Loss 101: Crunching Numbers

irst thing's first: weight loss is simple math—you must burn more calories than you consume. I know this might sound simple, but you'd be amazed at all the diets there are out there that cloud this issue. All of the members of my team on *The Biggest Loser* had tried countless diets, had stuck to it and avoided all the forbidden foods, and couldn't understand why they hadn't lost weight. Because, unbelievably, most diets, while they will tell you what you supposedly can and can't eat, do not deal with the cold, hard numbers. As everyone saw, my math seemed to work out for them when nothing else had. Let me break it down for you, too. Calories are a measure of the amount of energy provided by the food you eat—the more calories you eat, the more energy you are giving your body. If you give your body more energy than it can use, whatever you don't use will be stored as fat. In order to consume fewer calories than you burn and lose weight, you obviously first need to know how many calories your body is burning.

FIGURING OUT YOUR
ACTIVE METABOLIC RATE

The number of calories you burn in a day is known as your active metabolic rate (AMR). Rates vary from person to person, so it is crucial that you take the time to figure yours out—if you don't, you run the risk of consuming too many calories or even consuming too few. Both of these extremes are harmful: you don't want to take in energy that you don't use because it will be stored as fat, but you also don't want to take in too little energy or your body will start holding on to fat. Once you know your AMR, you will be able to balance caloric intake and expenditure in the way that's best for your weight-loss goals.

Your AMR takes into account the following three factors. You will need to make these three preliminary calculations in order to arrive at your total daily caloric expenditure.

1. Basal Metabolic Rate

Your basal metabolic rate (BMR) is the number of calories your body burns in a day when operating at absolute minimum capacity. Basically, if you sat on the couch all day long and did nothing, your BMR is how many calories your body would burn just to maintain basic activities such as heartbeat, digestion, respiration, and tissue repair.

Your BMR is influenced by a number of factors, among them age, weight, height, gender, environmental temperature, and your diet and exercise habits. The younger you are, the higher your BMR is likely to be, since younger people have higher rates of cellular activity. In addition, men will generally have higher BMRs than women, since men usually have a greater percentage of calorie-burning lean muscle tissue in their physical makeup. Because of these variations, it is hard to pin down your BMR to the exact calorie, but we can get close. Here are gender-specific formulas for figuring out your BMR, so get your calculator ready and plug your numbers into whichever formula applies to you.

MALE:
   66 + (6.3 × body weight in lbs.) + (12.9 × height in inches) - (6.8 × age in years)

FEMALE:
   655 + (4.3 × weight in lbs.) + (4.7 × height in inches) - (4.7 ×age in years)

Keep that calculator handy. Your basal metabolic rate only accounts for approximately 75 percent of your total daily caloric expenditure.

2. Daily Activity Level

The second factor in the calculation of your total daily caloric expenditure is how physically active you are in your everyday life, not counting exercise (that comes later). Determine which one of these descriptions best fits your day-to-day routine, then give yourself the appropriate score.

a. Sedentary Physical Activity Level
Do you have a desk job or do some other kind of work that entails sitting down for most of the day? If the answer is yes, your score is 1.1.

b. Light Physical Activity Level
Are you on your feet and walking around for half the day or more? Some examples of people who would fall into this category are stay-at-home mothers, salespeople, and doctors. If this is you, your score is 1.2.

c. Moderate Physical Activity Level
This level is if you're on the move pretty much all day, with a few limited periods of being sedentary. Ex-

amples of people in this category would be gardeners, carpenters, and mail carriers. If you're in this category, your score is 1.3.

d. High Physical·Activity Level

Does your job require being constantly on the move and does it entail significant amounts of manual labor? Examples of people in this category include construction workers, farm workers, and movers. If you're in this group, your score is 1.4.

Write down your daily physical activity level score here: _____

3. Exercise Expenditure

The third and final element you need to calculate your active metabolic rate is the number of calories you burn from exercise on an average day. The number of calories you burn during any exercise session depends on a few things, primarily your body weight. The one way *not* to figure out how many calories you burn during exercise is to go by the monitor on the machine you're using, since exercise machines are not set up to take everything into account and are generally inaccurate. The most effective way to calculate the calories you've burned during exercise is with a heart rate monitor. Once you've programmed it with your personal information, it will give you a much more accurate account of the calories you burn as you burn them. I cannot suggest strongly enough that you buy one. In the meantime, use the following chart to help you figure out the number of calories you burn from exercise on an average day according to your weight, the type of exercise you do, and its duration.

EXERCISE EXPENDITURE CHART

WEIGHT (in pounds)	100	125	150	175	200	225	250	275	300	325	350
ACTIVITY	CALORIES BURNED DURING 1 HOUR										
Walking 4 mph	199	249	299	349	399	449	499	549	599	649	699
Jogging 5 mph	376	426	476	526	576	626	676	727	776	826	876
Swimming	199	249	299	349	399	449	499	549	599	649	699
Cycling 13 mph	560	610	660	710	760	810	860	910	960	1010	1060
Heavy Aerobic	444	494	544	594	644	694	744	794	844	894	944
Light Weights	172	222	272	322	372	422	472	522	572	622	672
Intense Weights	392	442	492	542	592	642	692	742	792	842	892

Write the number here: _____

Now write the three numbers you've come up with here:

BMR = _____

× × = _____

Daily Activity Score = _____

+ +

Exercise Expenditure = _____

=

Active Metabolic Rate = = _____

Simply multiply your BMR by your Daily Activity Score, then add your Exercise Expenditure. Whatever you get from this final calculation is your magic number. Now that you know your AMR, let's figure out how to lose some weight!

SETTING WEIGHT-LOSS
GOALS INTO A TIMEFRAME

A pound of fat is equal to 3,500 calories. Using your AMR, you can calculate with great precision exactly how many calories you have to consume and burn in order to lose the number of pounds you want. If you want to lose 1 pound in a week, you will have to build up a caloric deficit of 3,500 calories over the course of that week, or a deficit of 500 calories daily. To lose 2 pounds in a week, you'll have to create a caloric deficit of 7,000 calories over the week, or 1,000 calories daily, and so on. Get the idea?

With this simple math you can set your weekly weight-loss targets. Contrary to popular belief, losing weight quickly is not unhealthy if you do it through proper nutrition and exercise, *not* through starvation. Obviously, if you have a personal or family history of cardiac disease, you should consult your doctor before starting any diet and fitness program. But in general there is absolutely no scientific evidence to suggest that losing weight fast is harmful to your heart in any way if it's done right. There is a minimal risk of gallstones from dropping weight too quickly through severe calorie restriction, but exercise and adequate fiber intake will prevent this problem.

Having said that, my personal recommendation is that you aim for 2 pounds a week, since anything more ambitious than that could lead to burnout or bingeing. Remember, this is about creating a healthy lifestyle and instituting changes you can live with forever, not crash dieting. Rome wasn't built in a day.

COUNTING CALORIES

Now that you know how to calculate the number of calories you can consume while losing weight, it's time to learn some simple methods for keeping a record of your intake so that you know how to stay on target. To get started, you will need:

1. A food journal
2. A kitchen scale and measuring cups
3. A calorie-counter book—make sure you get one that includes information on protein, fat, and carbohydrate contents

Start keeping a written record of absolutely everything you eat throughout your day, and be detailed. For example, don't just write down chicken. Write down how it was prepared and how much you ate. At first you should measure and weigh your food to figure out exactly how many calories you're consuming, and it is important to make sure you are always measuring raw; when food is cooked, it is more dense and has more calories. I know measuring everything can be tedious, but it won't take long for you to know by heart what a cup of milk looks like or how many ounces of chicken are in a small breast. Before you know it, you'll be eyeballing your portions like a pro. If you find yourself in a situation where you don't have the luxury of using your measuring equipment, here are some useful tips for assessing portion sizes using your hand.

- ◆ The size of your fist is roughly equal to a cup-size serving of cereal, wild rice, black beans, and so on.
- ◆ The size of your thumb is roughly equal to an ounce-size serving of cheese, and so on.
- ◆ The tip of your thumb is roughly equal to a teaspoon of olive oil or butter.
- ◆ The center of the palm of your hand, without fingers, is roughly equal to a 3-ounce serving of fish, chicken, beef, and so on.

At the end of every day, use your calorie-counter book to add up the calories you have consumed. There are even websites such as www.caloriesperhour.com that will add them up for you. Using these simple methods, you can make sure you are eating the right amount of calories to achieve your weight-loss goals.

HOW LOW CAN YOU GO

As you start to design a dietary plan based on your target weight, there are a couple of things it's good to know about calorie restriction and your metabolism. One of the keys to successful, continued weight loss is keeping your metabolism working at top speed so that you are burning as many calories as you can. When you start to eat less, however, your metabolism will slow down to conserve energy in reaction to the reduction in your caloric intake. This is what causes the dreaded dieter's plateau. We've all been there: you start off full of determination, but all of a sudden the pounds stop coming off. There is nothing more discouraging than stepping on the scale after a week of diligent dieting and grueling workouts, and not seeing any drop in the numbers. The plateau is a common problem among dieters and can typically be waited out. Stick with it for a few weeks and the scale will most likely continue its downward swing. But there are also measures you can take to try and keep your metabolism fired up even as you reduce your caloric intake.

To begin with, it is important never to let your caloric intake drop below 1,500 if you're a man and 1,200 if you're a woman. Restricting yourself any further will quickly signal your metabolism to slow down. Also, don't go too long without eating. Four hours without food is a reasonable maximum. Don't skip meals and always eat breakfast. This will keep your blood sugar stable and cravings under control.

Another way to prevent your metabolism from slowing is to vary your intake from day to day throughout the week—the human body cannot slow metabolism to adjust to a reduced caloric intake if it isn't fixed from one day to the next. For example, if I want to lose 1 pound in a week, I have to create a caloric deficit of 3,500 over the course of that week. My weekly AMR (my daily AMR multiplied by 7) is 13,300, so in order to lose 1 pound, I will have to limit my weekly caloric intake to 9,800 (my AMR minus the 3,500 calories that burn off 1 pound). As long as I don't consume more than 9,800 calories during the week, I will lose that pound, but rather than eating 1,400 calories each day to achieve that weekly deficit, I'm much better off varying intake from day to day so that my metabolism is not able to adapt to a fixed reduction. Here's an example of how I could break the numbers down:

Monday:	1,200 calories
Tuesday:	1,500 calories
Wednesday:	1,200 calories
Thursday:	1,600 calories
Friday:	1,200 calories
Saturday:	1,400 calories
Sunday:	1,700 calories
Total weekly caloric intake:	9,800

See how this works? My total weekly caloric intake is 9,800, which is where I need it to be in order to lose 1 pound, but I've varied my daily caloric intake so that my metabolism isn't able to adapt to the restriction.

There are also some exercise-based solutions to the dieter's plateau, which I will cover in the Sweat section.

The plateau effect can be a factor of plain and simple flagging resolve. If you've hit a plateau and mixing up your caloric intake just isn't working, make sure you are not slipping on your diet without realizing it and that you are not slacking off in your workouts. Make sure as well that you are keeping up with your food journal and that you are being honest and accurate. The bottom line when it comes to the dieter's plateau is this: It will pass. *Don't give up.*

One last thing to keep in mind as you begin: When you start a new diet and exercise program, you will lose a significant amount of water weight at first, and it's likely that in the first month you will lose more weight than you would ordinarily expect from the caloric deficits you are building up from week to week. By month 2, your system will begin to even itself out, and weight loss will continue at whatever rate is appropriate to your caloric intake/deficit ratios. Again, 2 pounds a week is a reasonable weight-loss goal, but now that you know how to work the numbers for yourself, you can design your regimen around any weekly weight-loss goal you like.

7

Metabolic Typing

You may be thinking that as long as you stay within your caloric range for the week, you can eat whatever you want. Although it's true that at a basic level weight loss is simple math, there is more to losing weight and getting healthy than just numbers. As you restrict your caloric intake, it is absolutely essential that you eat the right kinds of food to build muscle, strengthen your immune system, and stay energized throughout the process. Sounds simple, right? It would be, except that the way to do this is different for everyone.

DETERMINING YOUR METABOLIC TYPE

For many years nutritional science has taken a generic, overly standardized approach to health and weight loss. This is why there is no one diet that works for everyone. There was all that hype about the Atkins diet, but Kelly, one of my contestants on *The Biggest Loser*, lost just one pound in a month of sticking to Atkins. Because I know that we are all different and need to diet according to our specific body's characteristics, I was able to coach her to lose fifty-five pounds in three months. We were working together on the show, and she lost thirty-five more after that.

Why? Inherited genetics make each one of us unique, from the color of our hair right down to the way our organs function. This uniqueness extends to the way our cells convert nutrients into energy. In order to know how to get the most nutritional bang for your calorie buck, you need to understand your unique metabolic type. Once you do, you can begin to custom design your new dietary lifestyle around the foods that will help you achieve and maintain your ideal weight while also optimizing your physical energy, strength, and mental clarity.

Metabolic typing is really just fancy talk for figuring out how your body processes what you eat—more specifically, how your body deals with the three basic macronutrients in food: carbohydrates, proteins, and fats. Imagine that you are a furnace: your body takes the food you eat and burns it with oxygen to convert its caloric content into energy. This process is known as oxidation, and it's how the carb content in your food gets turned into glucose and released into the blood. When glucose is released into the blood, the pancreas is cued to release insulin to "clean" your blood of any sugar that is not being used by the body as energy and carry it to your cells, where it gets stored as fat. The fact that we all oxidize the nutrients in our food in different ways is the reason why a particular diet will work for one person and not for another. If you know more about how the nutrients in your food act on your system, you can avoid a lot of unnecessary pitfalls and really maximize your results as you continue on your journey toward total health.

Although rates can vary a lot from one person to the next, most people can be classified according to three basic groups:

1. Fast oxidizers
2. Slow oxidizers
3. Balanced oxidizers

Fast oxidizers burn through the nutrients in their food very rapidly, with the consequence that the carb content is broken down to glucose and released into the blood almost at once. This sudden increase in blood sugar triggers a rapid release of large amounts of insulin to clean away excess sugar, which is stored as fat in your cells. The more carb content in your food, the more energy will be available to your body right away, and the greater the chance that it will not be needed and get stored as fat. Insulin is a quick and effective blood-cleaner, and the dramatic leaps and falls in blood sugar levels that result from fast oxidation lead to the sugar crash effect. For a fast oxidizer, foods with high carb ratios cause fatigue and carb cravings as well as promote fat storage.

Fast oxidizers should eat foods with more proteins and fats in order to slow down their rate of oxidation and insulin release, and to better promote stable blood sugar and sustained energy levels.

Slow oxidizers burn through the nutrients in their food slowly and do not release the glucose from carbohydrates into the blood quickly enough, which means that they do not get converted into glucose, and energy production and availability are delayed.

A slow oxidizer should eat foods with higher ratios of carbs, since protein and fat slow the rate of oxidation and energy production even further.

Balanced oxidizers fall right in between the two. They require foods that have equal quantities of protein, fat, and carbs in order to optimally process, produce, and use the energy from their food.

Now that we have defined the different metabolic types, you're probably wondering how you're supposed to know what's happening in your blood every time you have a snack. Don't worry—there's a test, and you can take it right now, *and* all you need is a pencil and paper. The test is made up of a series of detailed questions that bear on everything from the foods you crave to the dryness of your skin. These questions cover such a wide range of physical attributes because scientists now believe that metabolic type, i.e., the way in which your body processes nutrients, is wired right into a part of your central nervous system that controls a host of other functions within your body. Consequently, if you take a closer look at some of the peripheral functions in your own body, they will shed light on your particular oxidative type and help you pinpoint your specific nutritional needs.

Oxidizer Test

For each of these questions, circle the response that best applies to you. You may not know the answer right off the bat—it may take a couple of days if you have to see a pattern, but really think about these questions and analyze how different foods affect your body and your moods. The better you know yourself, the greater your odds of achieving exactly the results you want.

In the morning, you
A. Don't eat breakfast.
B. Have something light like fruit, toast, or cereal.
C. Have something heavy like eggs, bacon or steak, and hash browns.

At a buffet, the foods you choose are
A. Light meats like fish and chicken, vegetables and salad, a sampling of different desserts.
B. A mixture of A and C.
C. Heavy, fatty foods like steak, ribs, pork chops, cheeses, and cream sauces.

Your appetite at lunch is
A. Low.
B. Normal.
C. Strong.

Your appetite at dinner is
    A. Low.
    B. Normal.
    C. Strong.

Caffeine makes you feel
    A. Great—it helps you focus.
    B. Neutral—you can take it or leave it.
    C. Jittery or nauseous.

The types of foods you crave are (sugar is not listed because everyone craves sugar when they are tired or run-down)
    A. Fruits, bread, and crackers.
    B. Both A and C.
    C. Salty foods, cheeses, and meats.

For dinner you prefer
    A. Chicken or fish, salad, and rice.
    B. No preference—choice varies daily.
    C. Heavier, fatty foods like pastas, steak, and
        potatoes.

After dinner you
    A. Need to have something sweet.
    B. Could take dessert or leave it.
    C. Don't care for sweets and would rather have
        something salty like popcorn.

The types of sweets you like are
    A. Sugary candies.
    B. No preference.
    C. Ice cream or cheesecake.

Eating fatty foods like meat and cheese before bed
    A. Interferes with your sleep.

B. Doesn't bother you.
C. Improves your sleep.

Eating carbs like breads and crackers before your bed
A. Interferes with your sleep, but they're better than heavier foods.
B. Doesn't affect you.
C. Is better than nothing, but you sleep better with heavier foods.

Eating sweets before bed
A. Doesn't keep you from sleeping at all.
B. Sometimes makes you feel restless in bed.
C. Keeps you up all night.

Each day, you eat
A. Two or three meals with no snacks.
B. Three meals with maybe one light snack.
C. Three meals and a lot of snacks.

Your attitude toward food is
A. You often forget to eat.
B. You enjoy food and rarely miss a meal.
C. You love food and it's a central part of your life.

When you skip meals, you feel
A. Fine.
B. You don't function at your best, but it doesn't really bother you.
C. Shaky, irritable, weak, and tired.

Your attitude toward fatty foods is
A. You don't like them.
B. You like them occasionally.
C. You crave them regularly.

When you eat fruit salad for breakfast or lunch, you feel
- A. Satisfied.
- B. Okay, but you usually need a snack in between meals.
- C. Unsatisfied and still hungry.

What kind of food drains your energy?
- A. Fatty foods.
- B. No food affects you this way.
- C. Fruit, candy, or confections, which give you a quick boost, then an energy crash.

Your food portions are
- A. Small—less than average.
- B. Average—not more or less than other people.
- C. Large—usually more than most people.

How do you feel about potatoes?
- A. You don't care for them.
- B. You could take them or leave them.
- C. You love them.

Red meat makes you feel
- A. Tired.
- B. No particular feeling one way or the other.
- C. Strong.

A salad for lunch makes you feel
- A. Energized and healthy.
- B. Fine, but it isn't the best type of food for you.
- C. Sleepy.

How do you feel about salt?
- A. Foods often taste too salty.
- B. You don't notice one way or the other.
- C. You crave salt and salt your food regularly.

How do you feel about snacks?
  A. You don't really snack, but you like something sweet if you do.
  B. You can snack on anything.
  C. You need snacks but prefer meats, cheeses, eggs, or nuts.

How do you feel about sour foods like pickles, lemon juice, or vinegar?
  A. You don't like them.
  B. They don't bother you one way or the other.
  C. You like them.

How do you feel about sweets?
  A. Sweets alone can satisfy your appetite.
  B. They don't bother you but don't totally satisfy you.
  C. You don't feel satisfied and often crave more sweets.

When you just eat meat (bacon, sausage, ham) for breakfast, you feel
  A. Sleepy, lethargic, or irritable.
  B. It varies day to day.
  C. Full until lunch.

When you eat heavy or fatty foods, you feel
  A. Irritable.
  B. Neutral—they don't affect you.
  C. Satisfied.

When you feel anxious
  A. Fruits or vegetables calm you down.
  B. Eating anything calms you down.
  C. Fatty foods calm you down.

You concentrate best when you eat
    A. Fruits and grains.
    B. Nothing in particular.
    C. Meat and fatty food.

You feel more depressed when you eat
    A. Fatty or heavy foods.
    B. Nothing in particular.
    C. Fruits, breads, or sweets.

You notice you gain weight when you eat
    A. Fatty foods.
    B. No particular food. You gain weight when
       you overeat.
    C. Fruits or carbs.

What type of insomnia, if any, applies to you?
    A. You rarely get insomnia from hunger.
    B. You rarely get insomnia, but if you do, you
       often need to eat something in order to fall
       back asleep.
    C. You often wake up during the night and need
       to eat. If you eat right before bed, it allevi-
       ates the insomnia.

Your personality type is
    A. Aloof, withdrawn, or introverted.
    B. Neither introverted nor extroverted.
    C. Extroverted.

Your mental and physical stamina are better when
you eat
    A. Light proteins like egg whites, chicken, or fish
       and fruits.
    B. Any wholesome food.
    C. Fatty foods.

Your climate preference is
    A. Warm or hot weather.
    B. Doesn't matter.
    C. Cold weather.

You have problems with coughing or chest pressure.
If yes, "C"; if no, move on to the next question.
You have a tendency to get cracked skin or dandruff
If yes, "C"; if no, move on to the next question.
You have a tendency to get light-headed or dizzy
If yes, "C"; if no, move on to the next question.

Your eyes tend to be
    A. Dry.
    B. Fine.
    C. Teary.

Your facial coloring is
    A. Noticeably pale.
    B. Average.
    C. Pink or often flushed.

Your fingernails are
    A. Thick.
    B. Average.
    C. Thin.

Your gag reflex is
    A. Insensitive.
    B. Normal.
    C. Sensitive.

You get goose bumps
    A. Often.
    B. Occasionally.
    C. Very rarely.

You are prone to
    A. Constipation.
    B. No stomach problems.
    C. Diarrhea.

When insects bite you, your reaction is
    A. Mild.
    B. Average.
    C. Strong.

Your body type is
    A. Short and stocky.
    B. Average.
    C. Tall and thin.

Your nose is
    A. Dry.
    B. Normal.
    C. Runny.

Scoring Your Metabolic Typing Test

When you have finished the test, add up the number of A answers, B answers, and C answers you have circled.

A_____ B_____ C_____

If your number of C answers is 5 or more higher than your number of A or B answers, you are a fast oxidizer.

If your number of A answers is 5 or more higher than your number of B or C answers, you are a slow oxidizer.

If your number of B answers is 5 or more higher

than your number of A or C answers, or if neither A, B, nor C's are 5 or more higher than the other two, you are a balanced oxidizer.

If you've answered this questionnaire and you are still not clear which category is the right one for you, there are two other tests you can take to help clarify your metabolic type. These tests are a little drastic and provocative, and they are only intended for those who truly cannot type themselves using the questionnaire.

1. **Niacin test:** Take 50 milligrams of niacin on an empty stomach. If you experience an immediate flush, you are most likely a fast oxidizer. If you experience a moderate flushing effect, you are a balanced oxidizer. If you experience a significantly delayed flushing or nothing at all, you are a slow oxidizer.
2. **Vitamin C test:** Take 8 grams of vitamin C in equally divided doses over 8 hours. The fast oxidizer will respond by feeling acidic and uncomfortable, and may even experience other symptoms such as diarrhea, nausea, or increased intestinal gas. A true balanced oxidizer may find that his or her stomach feels less acidic. A slow oxidizer will have no response at all.

I'm assuming you have now identified yourself somewhere along the fast-slow continuum. Now it's time to get to know more about your type. Read whichever section applies to you to learn the particular foods and eating habits that are right for your type. If you're good to your metabolism, it'll return the favor by working to help you maintain weight loss and good health.

FAST OXIDIZERS

Fast oxidizers

You require foods with higher percentages of protein and fat than carbohydrates. Make sure there is protein in everything you eat including snacks. Your ideal macronutrient ratio is 20 percent carbs, 50 percent protein, 30 percent fat.

Proteins

All proteins are not created equal. The ones that are best for you are high-purine proteins, which are commonly found in fattier meats. This is not to say that you should cut out chicken or fish, but you need the heavier proteins most because they help slow down your rate of oxidation. Choose from this list of proteins when deciding on a meal or snack.

> High Purine: organ meats (pâté, liver, etc.), herring, mussels, sardines, anchovies

> Moderate Purine: beef, bacon, dark meat chicken, duck, lamb, spareribs, dark meat turkey, veal, wild game, salmon, shellfish (lobster, shrimp, crab), oysters, scallops, octopus, squid, dark tuna

> Low Purine: cottage cheese, milk, yogurt, eggs, cheese, white meat chicken, turkey, fish

Carbohydrates

Your metabolism thrives when your carb intake is limited, but there are different kinds of carbs. Some aren't as bad as others. Avoid simple carbs, which convert to sugar quickly in the bloodstream. The carbs you can incorporate into your diet are the complex kind found mostly in nonstarchy vegetables. You can choose from these ideal carbs when deciding on a meal or snack.

> Low-Starch vegetables: asparagus, cauliflower, celery, mushrooms, spinach
>
> Fruits: avocado, olives, apples and pears (in limited quantity and never without protein on the side)
>
> Grains: sprouted grain bread only (Ezekiel bread is a well-known brand that is available at supermarkets and health–food stores)
>
> Legumes, tempeh, tofu

Fats

To best support your metabolism, you should be getting roughly 30 percent of your daily caloric intake from natural oils and fats. Choose these ideal fats when deciding on meal or snack preparation.

> Nuts/Seeds (listed in order of protein content): walnuts, pumpkin seeds, peanuts, sunflower seeds, sesame seeds, almonds, cashews, Brazil nuts, filberts, pecans, chestnuts, pistachios, coconut, macadamias
>
> Fat/Oils: butter, cream, almond oil, peanut oil, coconut oil, sesame oil, flaxseed oil, sunflower oil, walnut oil

Along with knowing the foods that are ideal for you, it is important to know the foods that are worst for you. You don't always have to eat off the ideal foods list, but the following foods will sabotage your weight-loss efforts.

1. Don't ever eat a meal that is predominantly carbohydrates.
2. Don't drink alcohol. It causes an increase in blood sugar and fat storage, and it will lead to a sugar crash as well as an increased appetite for carbs. If you choose to have a drink, avoid sugary cocktails, beer, and wine. Stick to clear alcohols like vodka or rum with calorie-free mixers like diet or club soda, and you can always just do what I do and drink it all straight.
3. Don't eat carbohydrates that are high on the glycemic load index. The next chapter will tell you everything you need to know about the GLI. For now all you need to know is to stay away from high-GLI foods. It is important for all metabolic types to watch their high-GLI intake, but it is especially crucial for you. If you should happen to eat high-GLI foods, make sure to combine them with a protein in order to slow down the production and release of blood sugar.
4. Don't drink too much caffeine. It is true that caffeine can be used as a fat burner and a performance enhancer when exercising. This is only effective, however, when the caffeine is taken in pill form in conjunction with aspirin. In the forms of coffee, tea, and soda, caffeine gives you short-term energy but does so by getting your adrenal glands to dump adrenaline into your blood like it's going out of style. As a result, when the caffeine leaves your system, your adrenal glands will be depleted for a while, which leaves you feeling weak and tired from substandard blood-adrenaline levels. Caffeine also speeds the rate of oxidation, which is the exact opposite of what you want your nutrients to do. Avoid caffeinated beverages whenever possible and keep your overall caffeine consumption to a minimum.
5. Don't overcook your meat. Avoid overcooked animal

products, since heat destroys essential amino acids and valuable enzymes.

You will have less physical ailments and feel energized if you eat the foods that contain the ideal macronutrient ratios for your metabolic type. However, these foods are all very high in calories. You must remember to keep within your caloric allowance in order to lose weight.

SLOW OXIDIZERS

In order to best serve your metabolism and feel energized both physically and mentally, you require foods with a higher percentage of carbohydrates. Your ideal macronutrient ratio is 60 percent carbs, 25 percent protein, and 15 percent fat.

Proteins

The best proteins for slow oxidizers are low-purine proteins, which are found in leaner meats. It's not that you can never have steak again, but high-purine, high-fat proteins slow down the rate at which you convert nutrients into energy, which is what you're already doing too slowly, so the less the better. In general, you want to stick to this list.

> Low Purine
> white meat chicken, turkey breast, lean pork, catfish, cod, flounder, perch, sole, trout, white meat tuna, swordfish, low-fat cheese, low-fat cottage cheese, skim milk, low-fat yogurt, egg whites

Carbohydrates

Although your metabolic type is better than the others at processing carbs, you still have to pick and choose carefully.

You want to avoid simple carbs, which convert into sugar very quickly in the bloodstream, and choose complex carbs instead. Follow this list of ideal carbohydrates when deciding on a meal or snack.

> Vegetables—Low Starch
> asparagus, cauliflower, celery, mushrooms, spinach, broccoli, brussels sprouts, cabbage, collard greens, cucumbers, garlic, kale, leafy greens, onions, peppers, scallions, sprouts, tomatoes, watercress

> Vegetables—Moderate Starch
> beets, eggplant, jicama, okra, yellow squash, zucchini

> Fruits
> apples, berries, cherries, citrus fruits, peaches, pears, apricots, plums, tropical fruits, olives

> Grains
> barley, brown rice, buckwheat, corn, couscous, kasha, millet, oat, quinoa, rye, spelt

> Legumes
> tempeh, tofu (eat sparingly as they are high in purines) beans, peas (should be eaten fresh, never dried)

Fats

You should be on a low-fat diet to keep your metabolism working smoothly. This does not mean no fat—fat is still an essential part of any healthy diet. You should allow 15 percent of your caloric intake to come from fat. You can go over that percentage if you like, but eating foods that are too high in fat content can make you feel lethargic, anxious, and irritable. Choose from this list of fats when cooking a meal or having a snack.

Nuts/Seeds
raw and unsalted only—be very sparing

Fats/Oils
vegetable or nut oils such as almond, coconut, flaxseed, olive, peanut, sunflower, walnut

It's not enough to know the foods that are ideal for you—you also have to learn which foods are worst for you. If you find yourself straying from the list of suggestions, remind yourself of these guidelines.

1. Don't eat foods that are fatty or that contain high-purine proteins, such as organ meats and fish such as herring and sardines. Limit your intake of fats and oils, as they will slow down your ability to convert food into energy even further. Avoid red meat or dark white meats, and stay away from high-fat dairy, nut butters, and avocados.
2. Don't drink alcohol. This is less of a concern for you than for fast oxidizers, but at the end of the day alcohol still increases your blood sugar and inhibits fat metabolism.
3. Don't drink too much caffeine. This too is less of a concern for you than it is for fast oxidizers, but caffeine gives you energy by acting on your adrenal glands, causing them to over-produce and flood your system with adrenaline. When the caffeine's effect has worn off, your adrenals are exhausted and you are left with lower-than-normal levels of adrenaline in your system, which makes you feel tired and sluggish.
4. Don't exceed one serving per meal of simple or starchy carbs like potato, pasta, or rice, and always eat them with a lean protein to help stabilize your blood sugar.

Remember to consume your ideal foods in accordance with your caloric allowance; otherwise, you will not lose weight.

BALANCED OXIDIZERS

If you are a balanced oxidizer, your diet is the easiest to follow, since you require an equal percentage of carbs, fats, and proteins. You feel at your best on a diet that incorporates a wide range of foods. Your ideal macronutrient ratio is 40 percent carbs, 30 percent protein, and 30 percent fat.

Proteins

You operate best when you are getting 30 percent of your total calories from protein. Be careful to mix the kinds of protein you eat so that you consume high-fat and high-purine proteins with low-fat and low-purine proteins. Choose from this list of proteins when deciding on a meal or snack.

High Purine
organ meats (pâté, liver, etc.), herring, mussels,
    sardines, anchovies

Moderate Purine
beef, bacon, dark meat chicken, duck, lamb,
    spareribs, dark meat turkey, veal, wild game,
    salmon, shellfish (lobster, shrimp, crab),
    oysters, scallops, octopus, squid, dark tuna,
    eggs, regular-fat cheeses

Low Purine
white meat chicken, turkey breast, lean pork,
    catfish, cod, flounder, perch, sole, trout,
    white tuna, swordfish, low-fat cheese, low-
    fat cottage cheese, skim milk, low-fat yogurt,
    egg whites

Carbohydrates

With regard to carbs, the real significant difference between balanced, fast, and slow oxidizers is not the types of carbs allowed but the quantity. You should get 40 percent of your nutrients from carbs, but like everyone you should avoid simple carbs and foods that are rated high on the glycemic load index, which we get into in the next chapter. Refined sugars like those found in cookies, sweets, and soda and processed grains like white bread or white rice should be shunned whenever possible, especially on a weight-loss regimen. You do best with a mix of fruits and vegetables from both the fast and slow oxidizers' carb lists.

Vegetables—Low Starch
asparagus, cauliflower, celery, mushrooms, spinach, broccoli, brussels sprouts, cabbage, collard greens, cucumbers, garlic, kale, leafy greens, onions, peppers, scallions, sprouts, tomatoes, watercress

Vegetables—Moderate Starch
beets, eggplant, jicama, okra, yellow squash, zucchini

Fruits
apples, berries, cherries, citrus fruits, peaches, pears, apricots, plums, tropical fruits

Grains
barley, brown rice, buckwheat, corn, couscous, kasha, millet, oat, quinoa, rice, rye, spelt

Legumes/Lentils (all fresh, nothing dried)
tempeh, tofu, beans, peas

Fats

In order to best support your metabolism, you need to be getting roughly 30 percent of your calories from natural oils and fats. Don't eat excessive amounts of fat, but don't specifically restrict your fat intake. You can choose from fats on both the fast and slow oxidizers' lists of permissible fats.

Nuts/Seeds (listed in order of protein content)
walnuts, pumpkin seeds, peanuts, sunflower seeds, sesame seeds, almonds, cashews, Brazil nuts, filberts, pecans, chestnuts, pistachios, coconut, macadamias

Fats/Oils
butter, cream, almond oil, peanut oil, coconut oil, sesame oil, flaxseed oil, sunflower oil, walnut oil

Eat the foods that are ideal for you. Also remember these guidelines of what not to do.

1. Don't eat meals made up of just one macronutrient. Make sure you adhere to your ideal ratio of 40 percent carbs, 30 percent protein, and 30 percent fat.
2. Don't drink alcohol. It depletes glycogen storage in the liver, which causes an increase in blood sugar and fat storage. In addition, you will most likely experience a sugar crash, which leads to a heightened appetite for carbs and the nutrients you need to metabolize them. If you do have a drink, choose wisely and avoid sugary cocktails, beer, and wine. Opt instead for clear alcohols such as vodka or rum with calorie-free mixers, like club soda diet, light fruit juices or diet Snapple. And there's always straight or on the rocks as well.
3. Don't eat foods that are high on the glycemic load index. (Again, see the next chapter for a full understanding of

glycemic load.) If you should happen to eat high-GLI foods, make sure you accompany them with protein in order to show down the rate of oxidation and stabilize blood sugar and energy levels.

4. Don't drink too much caffeine. Caffeine is only effective as a fat burner or performance enhancer when taken in pill form and combined with aspirin. In the forms of coffee, tea, or soda, caffeine gives you short-term energy but does that by signaling to your adrenal glands to dump all of their store out into your blood. When the caffeine wears off, your adrenal glands are so depleted they have to take a break, which means that you feel tired and weak.

5. Don't overcook your meat. Avoid overcooked animal products, since heat destroys essential amino acids and valuable enzymes.

Now that you have your list of foods that are ideal for your metabolic type, you will have more energy and feel better if you eat to support your metabolism. However, many of the foods on your list are high in calories. Your diet should incorporate these types of foods in accordance with your caloric allowance.

8

Carbs: The Good, the Bad, and the Glycemic Load Index

Now that you have identified your caloric allowance and the specific foods that are best suited for your particular metabolic type, you're ready for another major lesson: carbs. Don't panic—this isn't a program that demonizes all carbs. There is such a thing as a good carb, and there is room for good carbs in any wholesome, balanced diet. Once you understand which carbs you should avoid and why, you will be able to eat healthy and keep losing weight without being driven insane by the low-carb diet hysteria.

The difference between my program's nutritional recommendations and those of diets such as Atkins and South Beach is essentially a difference in carb evaluation. The Atkins and South Beach low-carb diets define carbs as good or bad according to the glycemic index, which is an incomplete rating based on how quickly the carb breaks down and releases glucose into your blood. Where these diets fall short is in only evaluating quality, not quantity, of carbs in any given food. I know this sounds confusing, but by only considering the *quality* of a given food's carbohydrate content, we do not get the whole story, and as a result these diets rule out many foods that actually belong in a healthy diet. The carrot is a perfect illustration of how the glycemic index can give a good food a bad name: the form of carbohydrate in a carrot turns into blood sugar quickly, which puts it high on the glycemic index and makes it a no-no for Atkins or South Beach dieters. However, if you step back to get a fuller picture, the total quantity of carbs in a carrot is low, which means that even though those carbs are turning into blood sugar quickly, there are so few that their overall effect on blood sugar is not very dramatic, so they are okay to eat.

By considering the quantity as well as the quality of carbs in any given food, you have a much more holistic and useful way of assessing its nutritional value—this more accurate and effective measurement is known as the glycemic load index (GLI). In this chapter you'll find a detailed glycemic load index table so that you will be able to make your own more informed, healthier food choices. The index pertains mainly to carbohydrates such as vegetables, fruits, and grains (because proteins and fats do not have much direct effect on blood sugar), and it is designed to help you figure out at a glance which carbs are okay and which you should avoid.

"Bad" carbs are the ones that get broken down in the body very quickly, triggering insulin release and promoting fat storage. If a food is high in bad carbs, it ranks high on the GLI, scoring 15 or higher. Bad or simple carbs often come in the form of refined sugars and processed grains; in fact, the reason that they break down so quickly in our bodies is that they have undergone chemical procedures during factory processing that are similar to the ones in our digestive system, so they are partially digested when we eat them. Pretty gross, huh? They are found in packaged foods such as white bread, pasta, crackers, baked goods, and other foods that are made with white flour and contain little or no fiber.

As if the sugar crash and fat storage promotion weren't

reasons enough to stay away from high-GLI foods, the rapid production of insulin has another adverse effect: When insulin levels in the blood increase, your blood drives amino acids into your muscles. When the concentration of an amino acid called tryptophan is increased relative to other amino acids, it is driven across the blood-brain barrier, where it interacts with a protein in the pleasure receptor area of the brain and stimulates the production of the pleasure hormone serotonin. This is why processed foods can become addictive both physically and psychologically— once you experience the pleasure effect from eating an unhealthy processed food, it is tempting to want to repeat the behavior again and again. The bottom line? Stay away from these carbs. They can sabotage you and will hold you back from achieving your fitness goals.

Good carbs—the ones that score 10 or below on the GLI—take a long time to digest, creating less of a need for immediate insulin release in the bloodstream and thus helping to stabilize your blood sugar level. They contain important vitamins, minerals, and nutrients that are essential for good health. Our bodies are genetically designed to consume these unrefined carbs such as vegetables and whole grains. They are often referred to as complex carbs due to their molecular structure.

Carbs that fall between 10 and 15 on the GLI are considered not optimal but not the worst thing in the world. Remember, these distinctions between good and bad carbs are important for *all* metabolic types. Even slow oxidizers who do best with higher ratios of carbs in their diet should be sure that they pick carbs from the lower end of the GLI. The following table of sample foods will help you identify and avoid the carbs that cause rapid blood sugar elevation, change brain chemistry, and trigger cravings. Be aware that you should not base your diet solely on the glycemic load index. It is important and valuable to be able to consider a food's GLI score as well as its caloric content, but there are foods that are low on the GLI and high in fat and calories.

Be conscious of your caloric allowance and stick to it. The GLI is just one more helpful tool in maximizing the success of your calorie-controlled, metabolically personalized weight-loss plan.

GLYCEMIC LOAD INDEX			
FOOD	SERVING SIZE	CALORIES	GL
Apple	1 medium	75	6
Apple juice	1 cup	135	12
Apricots	4 medium	70	6
Banana	1 medium	90	12
Barley	1 cup cooked	190	11
Black beans	1 cup cooked	235	8
Carrots	1 medium	30	3
Cashews	½ cup	395	4
Cherries	15 cherries	85	3
Corn chips	2 ounces	350	21
Corn on the cob	1 medium ear	80	17
Corn flakes	1 cup	100	24
Corn tortilla	1 medium	70	12
Cream of Wheat	1 cup cooked	130	22
Croissant	1 medium	275	17
French fries	6 ounces	515	25
Garbanzo beans	1 cup cooked	285	13
Grapes	40 grapes	160	13
Grapefruit	1 medium	75	5
Grapefruit juice	1 cup	115	9
Green vegetables	1 cup cooked	40	5
Ice cream	1 cup	360	10
Ice cream (low fat)	1 cup	220	13

Kidney beans	1 cup cooked	210	10
Kiwi	1 medium	45	6
Lentils	1 cup cooked	230	7
Macaroni and cheese	1 cup	285	46
Mango	1 medium	110	14
Milk (full fat)	1 cup	150	3
Milk (skim)	1 cup	70	4
Orange	1 medium	65	5
Orange juice	1 cup	110	15
Papaya	1 cup cut	55	9
Peach	1 medium	70	7
Peanuts	½ cup	330	1
Pear	1 medium	125	10
Peas	1 cup	135	3
Pineapple	1 cup cut	75	7
Pineapple juice	1 cup	130	15
Pizza	1 large slice	300	20
Plums	2 medium	70	4
Popcorn (full-fat)	2 cups	110	16
Potato (baked)	1 small	220	34
Potato chips	2 ounces	345	15
Pretzels	1 ounce	115	33
Pumpkin	1 cup mashed	85	3
Raisins	½ cup	250	42
Raisin Bran	1 cup	185	29
Shredded wheat	1 cup minisquares	110	15
Soda	16 ounces	200	33
Soda crackers	12 crackers	155	18
Soybeans	1 cup cooked	300	1

GLYCEMIC LOAD INDEX			
FOOD	SERVING SIZE	CALORIES	GL
Soy yogurt (full-fat)	1 cup	200	13
Strawberries	1 cup	50	1
Tomato juice	1 cup	40	4
Waffles	1 medium	150	18
Watermelon	1 cup cut	50	7
White bread	1 slice	80	20
White rice	1 cup cooked	210	23
Whole-grain bread	1 slice	80–120	14
Yam	1 cup cooked	160	13
Yogurt (full-fat)	1 cup	200	9

9

Good Fats versus Bad Fats

A long with understanding carbohydrates, it is useful to have a basic knowledge of fats. We have long been told fatty foods are high in calories and can lead to unhealthy levels of cholesterol and heart disease. But fat is also an integral part of a healthy diet, so it is key to know how to get the right kinds in the right amounts. Animal and vegetable fats provide valuable, concentrated energy; they also provide the building blocks for cell membranes and a variety of hormones and hormone-like substances. Fats slow down the absorption of nutrients into your system so that you can go longer without feeling hungry, and they aid in sugar and insulin metabolism, thus aiding in weight loss. In addition, they act as carriers for important fat-soluble vitamins, aid in the absorption of vital minerals, and help facilitate a host of other important biological operations within the body.

"GOOD FATS"

How do you know which fats are beneficial and which are toxic? Very basically it all boils down to molecular structure, and how the differently formed fat molecules affect your body. Let's start with the good fats: the fats considered to be healthiest come from plants and vegetables and are known as *unsaturated*. Unsaturated fat molecules contain at least one pair of carbons linked by a double-bond. Since hydrogen cannot break this bond and therefore cannot bond with all of the carbon present, any fat molecule with one or more double-bonded carbon is considered "unsaturated" by hydrogen.

Of the unsaturated good fats, the healthiest is *monounsaturated*, so named for its one pair of double-bonded carbons. This is the kind of fat that can actually lower your "bad" cholesterol and reduce your risk of heart disease. It also supplies fatty acids essential for skin health and cellular development, and is believed to help prevent certain kinds of cancer, including breast and colon cancers. Excellent sources of monounsaturated fat include olive oil, canola oil, nuts (raw, never roasted), and avocados.

Another healthful fat from the unsaturated family is known as omega-3 fat, which is a form of *polyunsaturated* fat, so named for its multiple pairs of double-bonded carbons. Omega-3 fats are found predominantly in cold-water fish such as salmon. They are also found in abundance in flaxseed, walnuts, and almonds. Like monounsaturated fat, omega-3 improves heart health by keeping cholesterol levels low, but it can also aid in stabilizing irregular heartbeat (arrhythmia) and reducing blood pressure. Omega-3 fatty acids act as natural blood thinners, reducing the "stickiness" of blood cells (or platelet aggregation), which can lead to blood clots and stroke. In numerous studies over the years, participants suffering from inflammatory diseases such as rheumatoid arthritis, lupus, and Raynaud's disease have reported less joint stiffness, swelling, tenderness, and overall fatigue when taking omega-3s. This fat may inhibit the production of carcinogens within the body, thus aiding in cancer prevention and cancer treatment. In addition, your brain, which is 60 percent fat, needs omega-3 to function properly. This wonder fat has even been shown to improve depression and symptoms of other mental illness.

Another group of fats that are now accepted as having health benefits are the *saturated* fats, which are found in meat, dairy, and other animal products. Saturated fat molecules are so-called because they are "saturated" with hydrogen, meaning their molecules contain as many hydrogen atoms as is chemically possible. Although they were once considered to be directly linked to coronary disease, the scientific evidence that once suggested adverse health effects has been overturned, and these fats are now considered important for many reasons, including their role in cellular development and hormone production, as well as their transport of many vital fat-soluble vitamins. As highly concentrated sources of protein and energy, saturated fat also helps slow down the rate at which you absorb food, therefore letting you go longer without becoming hungry again.

"BAD" FATS

Whereas the "good" fats are all natural animal or vegetable fats, bad fats are man-made. Trans-fatty acids or trans-fats as they are known are produced by the partial hydrogenation of oil. They are present in most processed foods like chips, margarine, cookies, and even breakfast cereals and protein bars, despite the fact that nothing in our food supply is more dangerous. The adverse effects of these toxins are still being discovered. They include contributing to cardiovascular disease by increasing "bad" and lowering "good" cholesterol levels, raising insulin levels in the blood and possibly leading to diabetes, and depleting your system of vital nutrients. They are also bad for the brain and nervous system.

Here's what the U.S. Food and Drug Administration has to say about it: "By our most conservative estimate, replacement of partially hydrogenated fat in the U.S. diet with natural unhydrogenated vegetable oils would prevent approximately 30,000 premature coronary deaths per year, and epidemiological evidence suggests this number is closer to 100,000 premature deaths annually."

Avoiding trans-fats can be tricky unless you know what to look for, since they are not currently listed as trans-fats on food labels. (New FDA guidelines forcing companies to disclose trans-fat content explicitly take effect in 2006.) Avoid products that contain hydrogenated or partially hydrogenated vegetable oils, or shortening. Processed foods that are commonly made with trans-fats include some margarines, baked goods, crackers, fried foods, salad dressings, to name just a few.

Now that you know which fats to avoid and which fats can be incorporated into a healthy diet, it is important to remember that just because a food is healthy does not mean it is also dietetic. Foods that are high in fat, good or bad, are high in calories, period. In order to shed those pounds and improve your overall health, you must adhere as closely as possible to your caloric allowance as well as to the list of foods recommended for your metabolic type.

10 | Food Labels: How to Decipher Them

N ow that you are empowered by knowing what to look for and what to avoid, an instrumental part of your success will be correctly reading food labels. The tips I will give you in this chapter will make it easier for you to do this so that you can make quick, informed food choices that contribute to your healthy diet. There are several things to look for on food labels.

CALORIES

First and foremost, you should be looking for the number of calories in any food you consume. Make sure you look at the serving size and the number of servings in the package. Calories are always listed per serving, not per container. Read the fine print on a small tub of ice cream, for example, and you'll discover that there are roughly 300 calories per serving and 4 servings per tub, meaning that this small tub has a total of 1,200 calories. Checking this information can be frustrating and confusing at first, but now that you know how to do it, you will never miscount calories again and can make changes so that you are in line with your personal calorie intake guidelines. Serving sizes are standardized and are measured in units we know such as cups or even pieces, which makes it easier to assimilate the nutritional information so that you are not squinting at labels for hours on end.

MACRONUTRIENT RATIO

The very next thing you should look for is the macronutrient ratio. You need to find out how many grams each of fat, carbs, and protein are in the food you are considering and make sure you are sticking to the ratio that is ideal for your metabolic type. Again it is important to be conscious of serving size and the number of servings per container, since these variables affect not only the calorie content but also the quantity of macronutrients you are consuming. Let's break down a sample label together.

What follows is a label for a box of macaroni and cheese. In this instance, the serving size is 1 cup, and there are 4 servings in the box. In 1 serving there are 320 calories, 160 of which—half—come from those 9 grams of fat. What if you ate the whole package? Four servings would mean 1280 calories, 640 of which would come from the total of 36 grams of fat. With almost 50 percent of its total calories coming from fat, the *degree* to which this food is damaging to your healthy diet will depend on your metabolic type. *However*, even if you are a fast or balanced oxidizer, and require higher percentages of fat in your diet, your ideal fat ratio is still only 30 percent, which means that the above food is high in fat, no matter how you look at it.

Finding the protein and fat contents of your food and measuring them against your ideal macronutrient ratio is relatively straightforward once you understand serving sizes. But figuring out a food's true carbohydrate content gets tricky. It might seem counterintuitive, but don't take the total number of carbs listed on the label at face value— the only thing relevant to us is the number of "net carbs" or "impact" carbs. The concept of net carbs is based on the fact

Boxed Macaroni and Cheese

Nutrition Facts

Serving Size 3.5 oz (98g/about 1/4 box)
(Makes about 1 cup)

Servings Per Container about 4

Amount Per Serving

Calories 320 Calories from Fat 160

	% Daily Value*
Total Fat 9g	14%
Saturated Fat 3g	15%
Trans Fat	0g
Cholesterol 20mg	7%
Sodium 820mg	34%
Total Carbohydrate 46g	15%
Dietary Fiber 2g	8%
Sugars 3g	
Protein 12g	14%

Vitamin A 2%	·	Vitamin C 0%
Calcium 10%	·	Iron 10%

*Percent Daily Values are based on a 2,000 calorie diet. Your daily values may be higher or lower depending on your calorie needs:

	Calories:	2,000	2,500
Total Fat	Less than	65g	80g
Sat Fat	Less than	20g	25g
Cholest	Less than	300mg	300mg
Sodium	Less than	2,400mg	2,400mg
Total Carb		300g	375g
Dietary Fiber		25g	30g
Protein		50g	65g

that certain carbs affect blood sugar levels and others don't. Fiber, considered a "nonimpact carb," is one that our bodies can't metabolize, and therefore it has no effect on blood sugar levels. Nonimpact carbs are thus subtracted from the total number of carbs so that you are only counting net. Let's look at a food label from a bag of whole-grain bread to illustrate this point.

Whole-Grain Bread

Nutrition Facts

Serving Size 1 slice (34g)

Servings Per Container 20

Calories 80

Calories from Fat 5

Calories from Saturated Fat 0

*Percent Daily Values are based on a 2,000 calorie diet.

Amount/serving	% Daily Value*	Amount/serving	% Daily Value*
Total Fat 0.5g	1%	Total Carbohydrate 14g	5%
Saturated Fat 0g	1%	Dietary Fiber 3g	10%
Cholesterol 0mg	0%	Sugars 0g	
Sodium 80mg	3%	Protein 4g	8%
Potassium 75mg	2%		

Vitamin A 0%	Vitamin C 0%	Calcium 0%	Iron 4%
Thiamine 8%	Riboflavin 2%	Niacin 6%	Vitamin B₆ 4%
Phosphorous 8%	Magnesium 6%	Zinc 4%	

As you can see, the total carb content is 14 grams, and the fiber content is 3 grams. After you subtract fiber from the total carb content, you are left with 11 grams of net carbs, which are the only carbs that matter for our purposes.

Many low-carb diets such as Atkins will tell you that sugar alcohols and other such carbohydrates are also non-impact carbs, but this is confusing. The misleadingly named "sugar alcohol," also known as polyol, is neither a sugar nor an alcohol but a man-made chemical compound with a molecular structure similar to that of sugars and alcohols. Food companies use it because it sweetens like sugar but is not counted as sugar according to FDA (Food and Drug Administration) guidelines.

Consequently, food companies can claim their product to be low in or free of sugar. Some companies even go so far as to subtract the sugar alcohol content from the carb count on the label, reasoning that it has a negligible effect on blood sugar levels when in fact this is not the case at all. Glycemic load values for the most commonly used sugar alcohols are certainly lower than for real sugars, but they are still significant and they do affect your blood sugar levels. As an example, take maltitol, a commonly used sugar alcohol with a glycemic value of 53, and compare it with corn syrup, a natural sugar derived from corn, with a glycemic value of between 85 and 92. Sure, maltitol's glycemic value is lower than the natural sugar, but it is still not low by any means. Bottom line: Sugar alcohols are impact carbs, and your body will use them as fuel or store them as fat, so you'd best include them in your net carb count. This can get tricky. Take a look at the example on the next page.

Protein Bar

	Amount/serving	% DV		Amount/serving	% DV
	Total Fat 7g	11%		Total Carbs. 19g	6%
	Sat. Fat 2.5g	13%		Dietary Fiber 8g	32%
	Trans Fat 0g			Sugars 1g	
	Cholesterol 0mg	0%		Sugar Alcohols 8g	
	Sodium 240mg	10%		Protein 14g	

Nutrition Facts

Serving Size 1 bar (50g)

Calories 170

Calories from Fat 70

*Percent Daily Values are based on a 2,000 calorie diet.

Vitamin A 35% · Vitamin C 100% · Calcium 50% · Iron 40% · Vitamin E 100% · Thiamine 100% · Riboflavin 100%
Niacin 100% · Vitamin B6 100% · Folic Acid 100% · Vitamin B12 100% · Biotin 100% · Pantothenic Acid 100%
Phosphorous 25% · Magnesium 40% · Zinc 40%

The label of this popular "low-carb" protein bar claims it contains a mere 2 grams of net carbohydrates. But look a little closer: the back label lists a total of 19 grams of carbs, which, if you look closer still, breaks down as follows: 8 grams of fiber, 8 grams of sugar alcohols, and 1 gram of sugar. But the sugar alcohol used in many of these products is maltitol, which you now know is in fact an impact carb. The only carbs in this product that will not actually affect your blood sugar levels are the 8 grams of fiber. So the true net carb count for this product is actually 11 grams, which is just under the net carb content of one slice of white bread, and certainly not as low as the packaging promises.

One more thing about sugar alcohols: they often produce a laxative effect. There are two reasons for this. First, they are not entirely absorbed into the body and tend to hold on to a lot of water in the bowel, which causes diarrhea. Second, when undigested carbs reach the colon, the normally present bacteria go wild with activity, which results in unpleasant bloating and gas.

FOOD LABEL TIPS

Here are some points to clarify common misconceptions about food labels.

1. Sugar-free does not mean carb-free. Compare the total carbohydrate content of a sugar-free food with that of a standard product. If there is a big difference in the carb content of the two foods, you may want to buy the sugar-free food. If there is little difference in the carb content of the two foods, choose according to taste and/or price.
2. "No-sugar-added" foods do not have any form of sugar added during processing or packaging and do not contain high-sugar ingredients, but they are not sugar-free. Check the label carefully. These foods may still be high in carbs.
3. Fat-free foods can be higher in carbs than their regular-

fat counterparts and may have almost as many calories. Fat-free cookies are a perfect example. Fat-free is not necessarily a better choice. Read your labels carefully.

4. If it seems too good to be true, it probably is. I had a client who one day mentioned that she used about a can of I Can't Believe It's Not Butter spray daily. When I proceeded to have a mild coronary, she was completely puzzled, because, as she protested, the packaging claims the product has 0 calories and 0 fat. Remember our little chat about serving sizes? It is true that per serving the product contains no calories and no fat, but the serving size indicated on the side of the can is "1 spray." The truth is that each serving could have as much as a ninth of a calorie or a ninth of a gram of fat, and the manufacturers would still be able to claim a 0 content. Per serving this seems like nothing, but who uses just 1 spray? All in all, the can actually contains 900 calories and 90 grams of fat! Yup, marketing people can be devious, so read the label. The ingredients list for I Can't Believe It's Not Butter spray includes several different oils, which is your tip-off that the 0 calorie–0 fat claim is totally false. Be cautious and keep yourself informed.

5. Ingredients are listed in descending order of predominance. If something is at the very end of the list, there is not very much of it in the food in question.

Along with having some basic label-reading skills, it's important to have some familiarity with all the terms and phrases that are assigned by the FDA and branded all over food packaging. Want to know the difference between "low fat" and "less fat," between "low sodium" and "very low sodium"? Allow me to shine a little light for you.

FDA SPECIFICATIONS FOR HEALTH CLAIMS AND DESCRIPTIVE TERMS

CLAIM	REQUIREMENT THAT MUST BE MET
Fat-free	Less than 0.5 g fat per serving, with no added fat or oil.
Low fat	3 g fat or less per serving.
Less fat	25% less fat than the regular-fat product.
Saturated fat-free	Less than 0.5 g saturated fat and 0.5 g trans-fatty acids per serving.
Cholesterol-free	Less than 2 mg cholesterol per serving and 2 g or less saturated fat per serving.
Low cholesterol	20 mg or less cholesterol per serving and 2 g or less saturated fat per serving.
Reduced calorie	At least 25% less calories per serving than the regular-calorie product.
Low calorie	40 calories or less per serving.
Extra lean	Less than 5 g fat, 2 g saturated fat, and 95 mg cholesterol per 100 g serving of meat, poultry, or seafood.
Lean	Less than 10 g fat, 4.5 g saturated fat, and 95 mg cholesterol per 100 g serving of meat, poultry, or seafood.
Light (fat)	50% or less of the fat than in the regular-fat food.
Light (calories)	One-third fewer calories than the regular-calorie food.
High-fiber	5 g or more fiber per serving.
Sugar-free	Less than 0.5 g sugar per serving.
Sodium-free, or salt-free	Less than 5 mg sodium per serving.
Low sodium	140 mg or less per serving.
Very low sodium	35 mg or less per serving.

FDA SPECIFICATIONS FOR HEALTH CLAIMS AND DESCRIPTIVE TERMS

CLAIM	REQUIREMENT THAT MUST BE MET
Healthy	Low in fat, saturated fat, cholesterol, and sodium, and contains at least 10% of the recommended daily values for vitamins A, C, iron, calcium, protein, or fiber per serving.
"High," "Rich in," or "Excellent Source"	20% or more of the recommended daily values for a given nutrient per serving.
"Less," "Fewer," or "Reduced"	At least 25% less calories or other nutrient per serving than the regular food.
"Low," "Little," "Few," or "Low source of"	An amount so insignificant that it allows frequent consumption of the food without exceeding the recommended daily values. This claim can only be made if it applies to all similar foods on the market.
"Good source of," "More," or "Added"	Provides 10% more of the recommended daily value of any given nutrient than the comparison food.

11

Tips and Recipes for Cooking Healthy at Home

I t's time to bring it all back home: Now that you know how to make healthy decisions at the supermarket, it's time to implement a few new habits in the kitchen. This will be simple, and don't worry, I won't have you eating cardboard or rabbit food. By following a few general rules, and making a few changes to your culinary routine, you'll find that you can lighten up most of the recipes you enjoy. Here is a list of tips and suggestions you can refer to (and refer to often) while cooking at home:

- ◆ Substitute Stevia or Splenda for sugar wherever possible. You can also use applesauce to sweeten cakes if you are baking.
- ◆ Use vanilla whey protein powder to replace the bulk of processed white flour in sweet baked goods. You can also try a 50-50 mix of protein powder and nut meal.
- ◆ Use nonstick cookware so that you can cut down on oils and butters and brown your foods using less fat. If you need oil, use it sparingly to cut down on calories.

Try cooking sprays like Pam or apply oil with a pastry brush so that you have as light a coating of fat on your food as possible.

◆ Replace fat-laden heavy cream or half and half with whipped evaporated skim milk. For best results, pour the canned evaporated skim milk into a metal mixing bowl. Place the mixing bowl along with your electric mixer's beater attachments in the freezer for about 30 minutes, or until ice crystals form around the edges. Remove the bowl and the beaters from the freezer; whip on high speed until soft peaks begin to form. Use at once.

◆ Use spices and lemon to flavor foods rather than fattening sauces or heavy, sugary marinades.

◆ Choose low-fat, low-cal, low-sugar, or low-carb versions of a food if they exist. Get low-fat dairy products like skim milk, low-fat cheese, and sour cream. Rethink all of your favorite condiments. Try out some low-cal, low-fat salad dressings until you find one you really like. Switch to fat-free mayonnaise and light variations of gravies and sauces. There are a wide range of low-carb condiments on the market including ketchups and barbecue and steak sauces. When you're cooking meat, choose the leaner cuts. Remove skin from chicken, but not until after cooking, so the meat will retain some of its moisture.

◆ Steam, bake, grill, braise, boil, or microwave your foods instead of frying them.

◆ When combined with water, bouillon cubes are a great low-cal way of adding robust flavor to most recipes that call for beef, chicken, or vegetable stock. You can also add bouillon cubes and water to stir-fries—they enhance the flavor and reduce the amount of fat needed to cook.

◆ Try using different vegetables as starch replacements. Spaghetti squash is great for replacing pasta, strips of zucchini or yellow squash can be cut with a shredder or vegetable peeler to replace lasagna noodles, and you can purée cauliflower as a stand-in for mashed potatoes. Be creative—the possibilities here are endless.

◈ When browning vegetables, put them in a hot pan, then spray with oil, rather than adding oil to the pan first. This reduces the amount of oil the vegetable can absorb during cooking.

You can use the above suggestions to transform recipes into healthier versions of old standby favorites, but you can also use them to come up with new dishes of your own. Be creative, think outside of the box, and you'll be astonished at how well you will be able to eat while still staying totally healthy. Just so you know I'm not lying to you, and so you can get your imagination going, I've included my favorite healthy—and delicious!—recipes for breakfast (on-the-go style and traditional sit-down), lunch, dinner, dessert, and snacks. Many of these won me major points with my team members on *The Biggest Loser*. But you needn't take our word for it, try them and see for yourself!

Breakfast

◆ French Toast

Serves 6; 100 calories per serving

1 egg white
1 cup half and half
1 tablespoon Splenda
1 tablespoon cinnamon
¼ teaspoon nutmeg
1 teaspoon orange or lemon extract
3 or 4 drops vanilla extract
¼ teaspoon salt
6 slices thick sprouted-grain bread
nonstick cooking spray
cinnamon and Splenda

In a wide bowl, beat the egg white with the half and half. Add Splenda, cinnamon, nutmeg, orange or lemon extract, vanilla extract, and salt. Dip each slice of bread in the mixture for a minute. Spray skillet with nonstick cooking spray and heat on medium. Cook french toast on both sides until brown. Dust with cinnamon and Splenda one last time and serve.

◆ Breakfast Burrito

Serves 4; 150 calories per serving

5 slices turkey bacon (nitrate-free)
nonstick cooking spray
6 egg whites, beaten
1 small tomato, cored, seeded, and chopped
½ cup low-fat shredded Cheddar cheese
4 six-inch low-carb tortillas
2 cups salsa for garnish

Place the bacon between two paper towels on a paper plate. Microwave on high 4–5 minutes, just until the bacon is crisp. Break into pieces. Spray a skillet with nonstick cooking spray and heat on medium. Scramble the egg whites in skillet until almost done. Add the tomato and bacon. Cook 30 seconds to 1 minute. Heat the tortillas for 10 seconds in the microwave, or you can warm them in a pan for a minute or two.

Spoon the egg scramble equally into center of tortillas. Sprinkle low-fat cheese on top. Fold burrito style. Serve immediately with salsa to taste.

◆ Asparagus Frittata

Serves 4; 100 calories per serving

½ tablespoon extra virgin olive oil
½ cup thinly sliced onion
1 clove garlic, minced
1 teaspoon chopped fresh thyme
12 cooked asparagus stalks, cut into 2-inch pieces
½ medium tomato, seeded and diced
1½ cups liquid egg whites
½ teaspoon salt
½ teaspoon pepper
½ cup freshly grated reduced-fat Parmesan cheese
nonstick cooking spray

Heat the olive oil over medium heat in a nonstick, ovenproof frying pan. Add the onion, garlic, and thyme. Sauté until the onion is soft but not brown. Add the asparagus and cook for a minute longer. Add half of the tomato and stir a few times. Remove the vegetables and wipe out the pan.

Turn on the broiler. In a mixing bowl, beat the egg whites, salt, pepper, and cheese together. Spray the same frying pan with nonstick cooking spray and heat on medium. Pour in the eggs and scatter the vegetables on top of the eggs. Turn the heat to low and cook 5–8 minutes until the frittata is golden brown on the bottom. Place the frittata under the broiler and cook until firm, about 5 minutes. Slide onto a plate and garnish with the remaining chopped tomato.

Frittatas make a nice, easy breakfast or handheld snack. They are adaptable too—you can add a spoonful of pesto or a few chopped sun-dried tomatoes to the egg mixture.

◆ Famous Red Team Puffs

Serves 1; 200 calories per serving

nonstick cooking spray
1/3 cup low-fat cottage cheese
2 egg whites
1 tablespoon Splenda
1 teaspoon unsalted butter
2 large strawberries, sliced
1 tablespoon chopped walnuts
2 tablespoons low-fat cream cheese, melted

Preheat oven to 350 degrees. Spray an individual tart pan lightly with nonstick cooking spray. To make the puff, blend the cottage cheese with the egg whites and Splenda, in a mixing bowl. Pour into the tart pan. Bake for 20–25 minutes. Remove the puff from the tart pan. Lightly grease a skillet with butter and heat on medium. Cook the puff with the sliced strawberries and chopped nuts until crisp. Drizzle melted cream cheese over the puff and strawberries and serve immediately.

Lunch

◆ Broccoli and Cheese Crustless Quiche

Serves 6; 150 calories per serving

nonstick cooking spray
12 egg whites, beaten
1 cup light sour cream
8 ounces shredded low-fat Cheddar cheese
10-ounce package frozen chopped broccoli, thawed,
    drained, and pressed dry
½ teaspoon black pepper

Spray a slow cooker with nonstick cooking spray. In a large mixing bowl, combine the egg whites, sour cream, cheese, broccoli, and pepper, then add to the slow cooker. Cover and cook on low 4 hours.

◆ Albacore Tuna Melt

Serves 4; 125 calories per serving

¼ cup fat-free mayonnaise
2 tablespoons coarsely chopped basil leaves
8 cloves roasted garlic, coarsely chopped
⅔ cup grated Asiago cheese
4 6-ounce pieces albacore tuna
extra virgin olive oil
salt and pepper to taste
1 ripe tomato, seeded and finely diced

In a medium mixing bowl, combine the mayonnaise, basil, garlic, and Asiago cheese together. Season the tuna on both sides with the olive oil, salt, and pepper. Heat a heavy frying pan on high until almost smoking. Add the tuna in a single layer and sear until lightly brown on one side. Turn with a spatula and sear the other side, about 2 minutes each side. The tuna should remain rare. Preheat the broiler. Spread the cheese mixture evenly over each piece of tuna. Broil 4 inches from the heat until the cheese bubbles. Sprinkle with the tomato and serve immediately.

◆ Cauliflower and Goat's Cheese Purée (Faux Mashed Potatoes)

Serves 4; 75 calories per serving

½ large head cauliflower, cored and cut into
    1-inch pieces
salt to taste
2 tablespoons fat-free whipping cream
2 tablespoons unsalted butter
2 tablespoons freshly grated reduced-fat
    Parmesan cheese
2 tablespoons reduced-fat goat's cheese

Cook the cauliflower over medium heat in a large pot of lightly salted water until completely tender, 20–30 minutes. Drain the cauliflower into a colander. With a bowl or small plate, press on the cauliflower to remove all the water. Toss the cauliflower and continue pressing. This step is very important to the texture of the dish. Transfer the cauliflower to a food processor. Add the whipping cream and purée until completely smooth. If you like a chunkier texture, mash by hand, adding the cream after the cauliflower is mashed. Return to the pot, heat on low heat, and stir constantly. Add the butter, Parmesan, and goat's cheese. Stir until blended and season with salt if necessary.

Serve immediately.

◆ Feta and Olive Meatballs

Serves 4; 200 calories per serving

½ cup chopped parsley
2 tablespoons finely chopped onion
1 pound lean ground lamb or beef
½ cup extra-nonfat crumbled feta cheese
⅓ cup pitted green olives, coarsely chopped
3 egg whites
2 tablespoons Tabil Spice Mixture (see below)
or 1 teaspoon dried oregano

Preheat the broiler.

In a large mixing bowl, combine all the ingredients with your hands and shape into 16 meatballs about the size of a silver dollar. Place the meatballs about 2 inches apart on a baking sheet and broil about 3 inches away from the heat until browned on top, about 5 minutes. Turn over and broil on the other side for about 5 minutes. You don't really need any salt in this recipe, as the feta and olives provide enough. Try the spice mixture. It tastes great in the meatballs. If you like, you can purchase low-carb tomato sauce to put over the meatballs.

◆ Tabil Spice Mixture

1½ tablespoons caraway seeds
¼ cup coriander seeds
2 dried red chilies

Roast the spices in a dry nonstick frying pan over medium heat until fragrant, about 2 minutes. Cool and finely grind in a spice mill.

Dinner

◆ Mexican Lasagna

Serves 12; 200 calories per serving

> 1½ pounds extra-lean ground beef
> salt and pepper to taste
> 1.25-ounce package taco seasoning mix
> 15 ounces low-fat ricotta cheese
> ¼ cup low-fat sour cream
> 27 ounces canned whole green chilies (drain and reserve
>   2 tablespoons canned juice)
> 2 tablespoons Tabasco sauce
> 4 six-inch, low-carb tortillas

Preheat oven to 350 degrees. Season the meat with a little salt and pepper. In a skillet over medium heat, break up the meat with a wooden spoon, and cook until browned. Drain off the grease. Stir in the taco seasoning mix and enough water to make a paste. In a small mixing bowl, whisk the ricotta cheese, sour cream, reserved chili juice, Tabasco, and ½ cup water. Spread a little of the mixture to cover the bottom of a 13 by 9-inch baking pan. Cover the sauce with a layer of tortillas, overlapping slightly. Sprinkle the meat mixture evenly over the entire base. Cover with a single layer of whole green chilies and pour the remaining sauce on top. Bake 45–60 minutes. Remove from the oven and allow to stand 5 minutes before serving.

◆ Texas Chili

Serves 6; 300 calories per serving

> 3 pounds chuck beef stew meat, fat trimmed, cubed
> 1 tablespoon minced garlic

¼ cup chili powder
1 teaspoon red pepper flakes
2 tablespoons quick-cooking tapioca
1 tablespoon oregano
1 teaspoon cumin
2 cubes beef bouillon
1 teaspoon black pepper
14½-ounce can fat-free beef broth
½ medium onion, finely chopped

Add all ingredients to a slow cooker and mix well. Cover and cook on low 8 hours. Stir chili well before serving. Sprinkle low-fat Cheddar cheese on top if desired.

◆ Crawfish Quesadillas

Serves 6; 200 calories per serving

1 medium onion, diced
1 medium bell pepper, diced
1 teaspoon extra virgin olive oil
1 pound crawfish meat without shells, drained

salt and pepper to taste
6 six-inch low-carb tortillas
2 cups shredded low-fat Cheddar and Jack cheese mix
6 tablespoons low-fat sour cream
2 medium tomatoes, diced

Preheat oven to 350 degrees.

In a skillet over medium heat, sauté the onion and pepper in 1 teaspoon of olive oil until tender. Add the crawfish and cook 5 minutes. Add salt and pepper. Spread crawfish mixture evenly across 3 of the tortillas. Sprinkle the cheese mixture evenly on top of the crawfish mixture and top each with another tortilla. Bake in oven for 10 minutes. Cut into four pieces and garnish with the sour cream and tomatoes.

◆ Veggie Pasta

Serves 4; 150 calories per serving

> 2 pounds spaghetti squash, halved lengthwise
>   and seeded
> 2 tablespoons extra virgin olive oil
> 1 red onion, sliced
> 1 zucchini, diced
> 1 yellow squash, diced
> 3 tomatoes, diced
> 1 clove garlic, minced
> ½ red pepper, diced
> ¼ teaspoon salt
> ¼ teaspoon pepper
> ½ cup freshly grated reduced-fat Parmesan cheese

Place the spaghetti squash halves, cut sides down, in a glass baking dish. Add ¼ cup water and cover with plastic wrap. Microwave on high 10 minutes until tender. Meanwhile, heat 1 tablespoon of the olive oil in a large skillet. Add the onion and cook over medium heat 3 minutes. Add the zucchini and yellow squash and cook 4 minutes. Add the tomatoes, garlic, and red pepper. Reduce heat and let simmer 10 more minutes. Using a fork, scrape the spaghetti squash strands into a bowl. Toss with the remaining tablespoon of olive oil. Spoon the spaghetti squash into the center of 4 pasta bowls. Pour the vegetable mixture over the top. Season to taste with salt and pepper. Garnish with low-fat Parmesan cheese as desired.

◆ Veggie Pasta with Italian Chicken Sausage

Serves 2; 492 calories per serving

> 2 small zucchini
> 2 tablespoons extra virgin olive oil
> Salt and pepper, to taste

1 garlic clove, diced
1 cup diced tomatoes
1 teaspoon oregano
½ pound cooked Italian chicken sausage, sliced into
    small pieces
¼ cup grated Parmesan, to taste

Using a vegetable peeler and turning as you go, slice zucchini into ribbons. In a skillet, over medium heat, sauté zucchini in 1 tablespoon of oil until soft and edges are clear. Add salt and pepper to taste. Over medium heat, heat 1 tablespoon of oil in another pan, and add garlic. Sauté for a minute, and then add the tomatoes and oregano. Simmer for a few minutes, and then stir in the sausage. Spoon sauce over zucchini. Sprinkle with Parmesan to taste.

◆ Chicken Parmesan

Serves 2; 500 calories per serving

½ cup crushed pork rinds
1 tablespoon oregano
1 tablespoon garlic powder
1 tablespoon grated low-fat Parmesan
3 egg whites
4 skinless, boneless chicken breasts
Nonstick cooking spray
1 cup tomato sauce (sugar-free marinara sauce)
2 cups shredded low-fat mozzarella

Preheat oven to 350 degrees.
    In a shallow bowl, mix rinds with spices and Parmesan. In another bowl, beat egg whites. Dip each chicken breast in egg white, then roll each breast in the rind mixture. Lay breasts in a baking dish coated with nonstick cooking spray. Bake 35 minutes. Add about ¼ cup tomato sauce over each breast and sprinkle each with about ½ cup mozzarella.

Return the dish to the oven and bake an additional 10 minutes or until chicken is no longer pink.

◆ Spinach Casserole

Serves 12; 80 calories per serving

1 bag (16 ounces) frozen spinach
7 cups fat-free cottage cheese
4 egg whites
1 pack (8 ounces) of reduced-fat feta cheese, crumbled
1 tablespoon onion flakes
½ cup grated reduced-fat Parmesan cheese

Preheat oven to 375 degrees.

Defrost and drain spinach. In a bowl, mix spinach with cottage cheese, egg whites, and feta. Add onion flakes to taste. Pour mixture into a 16 by 12-inch baking dish and sprinkle top with Parmesan. Cook for 45 minutes, until golden brown on top.

◆ Crab Stuffed Zucchini

Serves 2; 230 calories per serving

2 medium zucchini
6½-ounce can crabmeat, drained
1 ounce nonfat cream cheese, softened
¼ cup chopped onion
½ medium tomato, seeded and chopped
½ teaspoon lemon juice
1 tablespoon low-fat mayonnaise
dash liquid smoke
1 cup shredded low-fat mozzarella
nonstick cooking spray

Preheat oven to 350 degrees.

Discard ends of zucchini and cut in half lengthwise. Microwave for 3 minutes. Scoop out pulp, leaving zucchini shells. Chop pulp and mix with remaining ingredients; use only ½ cup mozzarella. Place zucchini shells in a baking dish coated with nonstick cooking spray and fill each with crabmeat mixture (it will overflow the shells). Top with rest of mozzarella and bake 20 to 30 minutes, until mozzarella is lightly browned.

◆ BBQ Pork Tenderloin

Serves 2; 230 calories per serving

    1 cup tomato sauce
    3 tablespoons Worcestershire sauce
    1 tablespoon vinegar
    1 teaspoon liquid smoke
    3 packets Splenda
    ¾ pound pork tenderloin
    salt and pepper, to taste
    Old Bay seasoning
    1 teaspoon extra virgin olive oil

In a small saucepan, combine tomato sauce, Worcestershire sauce, vinegar, liquid smoke, and Splenda, and cook over low heat for 10 minutes. As sauce cooks, cut the pork in ¾" slices and pound until thin. Sprinkle with salt, pepper, and Old Bay seasoning. Heat oil in a skillet. Sauté pork in oil a few minutes until nicely browned. Remove pork from pan, and pour sauce over the top of the tenderloin.

Dessert

◆ Crustless Cheesecake

Serves 12; 100 calories per serving

nonstick cooking spray
24 ounces low-fat cream cheese
1 cup low-fat ricotta cheese
½ cup low-fat sour cream
1½ cups Splenda
¼ cup heavy cream
1 tablespoon vanilla extract
1 tablespoon fresh lemon juice
5 egg whites

Preheat oven to 450 degrees. Spray a springform pan with nonstick vegetable oil cooking spray. In a shallow roasting pan big enough to fit the cake pan, pour in about 1 inch water and place on the center oven rack to preheat. In a large mixing bowl, beat the cream cheese, ricotta, sour cream, and Splenda just until blended. In a separate bowl, whisk the cream, vanilla, lemon juice, and egg whites until blended. Blend the egg mixture into the cream cheese mixture. Pour the batter into the greased springform pan. Place the pan into the heated water bath. Bake 15 minutes, then lower temperature to 275 degrees. Continue baking 1½ hours. Turn the oven off when done and leave the cake in the oven to cool 3 more hours. Remove the cake and refrigerate before serving.

◆ Apple Sour Cream Pie

Serves 8; 150 calories per serving

For the Meringue Crust
2 eggs whites
¼ teaspoon cream of tartar
¼ teaspoon salt
½ teaspoon vanilla extract
½ cup Splenda

Preheat oven to 300 degrees. In a large mixing bowl, beat the egg whites, cream of tartar, and salt until soft peaks form. Add the vanilla, and slowly beat in the Splenda until very stiff and glossy. Spread the mixture into a 10-inch pie plate to form a shell. Bake 50 minutes. Turn the oven off, and leave the meringue crust in the oven 1 hour so it cools slowly.

For the Filling
4 egg whites or ½ cup egg substitute
1/3 cup Splenda
2 tablespoons flour
1/8 teaspoon salt
1 cup low-fat sour cream
2 tablespoons fresh lemon juice
1½ pounds tart apples such as Granny Smith, peeled,
    cored, and sliced very thin
1/8 teaspoon ground nutmeg
butter-flavored cooking spray

Preheat oven to 400 degrees. In a medium mixing bowl, blend the egg whites or egg substitute, Splenda, flour, salt, sour cream, and lemon juice. Gently fold in the sliced apples. Pour into the meringue crust pie pan. Sprinkle with the nutmeg and coat with the entire pie with the cooking spray. Bake 40 minutes or until the top is browned and set. Chill before serving.

◆ Chocolate Chip Cookies

Makes 3 dozen cookies, 80 calories per cookie

- ½ cup (1 stick) butter
- ½ cup Splenda
- 2 large egg whites
- 1 teaspoon vanilla extract
- 1 cup vanilla whey protein powder
- 3 tablespoons unsweetened Hershey's Cocoa
- ½ teaspoon baking soda
- ⅛ teaspoon salt
- 2 tablespoons skim milk
- ¼ cup semisweet chocolate minichips

Preheat oven to 375 degrees. In a medium mixing bowl, beat the butter and Splenda until well blended. Add the egg whites and vanilla extract; beat well. In a separate bowl, stir together the protein powder, cocoa, baking soda, and salt. Add slowly to the butter mixture, pouring milk in simultaneously and beating until well blended. Stir in the chocolate minichips. Drop by teaspoonfuls onto an ungreased baking sheet. Bake 7–9 minutes or just until set. Remove from baking sheet to wire rack. Cool completely.

◆ Tiramisu

Serves 10; 150 calories per serving

For the Cake
nonstick cooking spray
4 ounces ground almonds
1 teaspoon baking powder
¼ teaspoon salt
6 eggs
½ cup Splenda
1 teaspoon vanilla extract

Preheat oven to 350 degrees. Spray a 15 by 10 by 1-inch pan with nonstick cooking spray. Line the pan with parchment paper and spray again with nonstick cooking spray. In a medium mixing bowl, combine the almonds, baking powder, and salt. Separate the eggs. In another medium mixing bowl, beat the egg yolks and Splenda with an electric mixer until thick and lemon colored, 3–4 minutes. Beat in the vanilla. Fold in the almond mixture. In a small mixing bowl, beat the egg whites to firm peaks. Stir one quarter of the egg whites into the almond mixture. Fold in two thirds of the remaining egg whites until barely combined, then the remaining egg whites until thoroughly combined. Spread evenly into the prepared pan. Bake 20–25 minutes until the top springs back when pressed lightly. Let cool.

For the Filling:
5 eggs
5 tablespoons Splenda
2 8-ounce containers mascarpone
½ cup strong coffee
3 tablespoons rum
½ cup unsweetened cocoa

Separate the eggs. In a medium mixing bowl, beat the egg yolks with the Splenda until thick and lemon colored. Add the mascarpone and beat it into the yolk mixture on low speed, scraping down the bowl. Do not overbeat or the mixture will curdle. In another medium mixing bowl, beat the egg whites to soft peaks. Stir one quarter of the egg whites into the mascarpone mixture. Fold in the remaining three quarters. Choose a large straight-sided dish such as a soufflé dish for assembling the tiramisu. Cut the almond cake into 16 fingers by cutting in half crosswise, then lengthwise. Cut each half crosswise into 8 fingers. Combine the rum and coffee in a shallow dish. Place the cocoa in a sieve over a bowl. Sprinkle the bottom of the dish lightly with cocoa. Quickly dip a few of the fingers into the coffee mixture and line the bottom of the dish. Do not get them too wet or your tiramisu will be runny. Spread on one quarter of the mascarpone mixture and dust the top with cocoa. Repeat the process until you have 3 or 4 layers. End with a sprinkling of cocoa. Cover and refrigerate overnight.

Snacks

◆ Cream Cheese Rollups

Serves 1; 80 calories per serving

> 2 tablespoons low-fat cream cheese
> 1 teaspoon cinnamon
> 1 teaspoon Splenda
> 1 six-inch low-carb tortilla

In a small mixing bowl, thoroughly combine the cream cheese, cinnamon, and Splenda. Spread on the tortilla. Roll up and enjoy.

◆ Smokey Buffalo Jerky

Makes 35 pieces; 30 calories per piece

> 1½ pounds pound buffalo tip roast
> 1 teaspoon liquid smoke
> 1 teaspoon garlic powder
> ¼ cup soy sauce
> 1 teaspoon pepper
> 1 teaspoon onion powder
> ¼ cup Worcestershire sauce

Slice the meat into quarter-inch strips. In a small mixing bowl, whisk the rest of the ingredients together and place in a zip-lock bag with the meat. Marinate for several hours at room temperature. Place on a clean oven rack with a baking sheet on a lower rack to catch drips. Do not overlap the meat strips. Heat oven to 125 degrees and cook 8 hours with the oven door slightly open. Check frequently so that meat doesn't get overdry.

◆ Spicy and Cheesy Toasted Pumpkin Seeds

Makes 2 cups; 150 calories per ½ cup

- 1 tablespoon egg white
- ⅛ teaspoon salt
- ¼ teaspoon cayenne pepper
- ¼ teaspoon garlic powder
- 2 teaspoon soy sauce
- ¼ cup very finely and freshly grated reduced-fat Parmesan cheese
- 2 cups raw, hulled pumpkin seeds

Preheat oven to 350 degrees. In a small mixing bowl, beat the egg white with a whisk until soft and foamy. Except for the pumpkin seeds, add the rest of the ingredients and combine thoroughly. Spread the pumpkin seeds in an even layer on a parchment-lined baking sheet. Coat with the egg white mixture. Bake 13–15 minutes until the pumpkin seeds pop. Let them cool completely and store in a covered container.

12 | Eating Out

As well as keeping it healthy on the homefront, it's important to know how to keep up your good work when you are out to eat. Many of my clients tell me that they have enormous trouble keeping to a healthy, nutritious diet when they go to a restaurant. I'm telling you right now—eating out is no excuse to fall off the wagon. And I don't want to hear that eating healthy when eating out is too expensive either—you could take me to any chain restaurant and I would still be able to stick to my diet. You *can* go about your normal life and still stay on track. The key to success is implementing a few new habits to arm yourself against temptation and make you sabotage-proof in any situation.

DINING ADVICE

1. Know your enemies and try to avoid them. It goes without saying that you should try and pick the healthiest restaurant possible, but if this isn't an option, identify ahead of time what things at the restaurant could throw you off your diet. Eliminate or address them in advance. If there is a restaurant that has a certain unhealthy food you know you can't resist, like the best french fries in

town, pick another place. There's always another restaurant. If you can't go healthy, go for variety so that if your kids are hell-bent on pizza, you might still be able to get salad, chicken, or fish.

2. Practice your environment control. Remember, willpower is way overrated, and you cannot eat what isn't there. If you are eating at a place that serves bread or chips on the table, ask the server not to bring them.

3. Get support. If you are with friends and they want the nachos supreme, recruit them to help you out. This goes back to chapter 3 on building your support system. Make your friends aware that you are watching what you eat, and ask them to help you resist. Have them keep the chips away from you, on the other side of the table, and tell them not to let you have any, no matter what.

4. Ask you server questions and educate yourself about the food so that you can make healthy choices. How is the food cooked, what's used in the preparation, what comes on the side—these are all things you want to know now that you are eating right.

5. Make substitutions. I'm always ordering the chicken fajita, but instead of the Mexican rice and refried beans, I ask for a salad on the side. Ask for grilled vegetables instead of a baked potato or french fries. Switch the hash browns for sliced tomatoes. You get the idea—this stuff will take a little extra thought at first, but in no time it'll be second nature.

6. Make modifications. If you have scoured the menu and there are no healthy options, you can usually create your own by requesting a few modifications to the preparation of your food. Ask if you can have your fish grilled instead of breaded; ask if you can have Dijon mustard sauce on the chicken instead of cream sauce; ask for the salad dressing on the side; get your omelet with egg whites; ask for the chef to use a small amount of olive oil.

7. Always hold the condiments or have them on the side. A healthy chicken salad that would be 300 calories can

quickly double if a fatty dressing is added to it. A burger can have up to 200 calories just from the ketchup you eat with it. Ask for your turkey sandwich with mustard instead of mayo. And here's another trick: bring your own condiments with you so that you are never stuck with what's available. I always bring my own low-calorie salad dressing when I go out to dinner. I've even gone so far as to bring my own low-calorie sugar-free barbecue sauce to a restaurant. If I do it, so can you!

8. Watch your portions. The portions we get in restaurants are for the most part completely out of control. Remember the ways to measure foods using your hand? Use them to make rough assessments. Make sure you don't go overboard just because there's more food on your plate than you need. Share an entrée with a friend, or ask the server to put half your meal in a doggy bag before he even brings it to the table so that you can save it for lunch the next day.

9. Fill up on fiber. Eat as many veggies and as much salad as you can (as long as the dressing is on the side!), because this will make you feel more full and keep you from overeating other, more fattening foods.

10. Don't feel guilty for leaving food on your plate. Stop eating if you are full. Ask the server to take away your plate. If you have to get extreme, you can even destroy the food by dumping salt all over it—get creative about empowering yourself to beat temptation before it beats you.

11. Be social. There are exceptions, of course, but in general dining out should be a pleasurable experience that revolves around more than just food. Sit back, relax, enjoy the company, eat slowly, and savor the whole experience.

THE BEST RESTAURANT OPTIONS

Let's get a little more specific. Here is a guide for the healthiest options at different kinds of restaurants so that you can stay on target.

Mexican

Chicken, beef, or shrimp fajitas with black beans or salad on the side instead of rice; carne asada (steak with onions and peppers); shrimp diablo (this is grilled with garlic butter—ask them to go easy on that); grilled fish tacos (with one corn tortilla rather than two); taco and tostada salads with chicken, beef, or shrimp for protein (don't eat the taco bowl). Get everything à la carte. Don't get the rice and only eat the beans if they are not refried.

Chinese

Any dish that isn't breaded and deep-fried. Avoid rice and noodles. Try and steer clear of sugar sauces like sweet and sour. Opt for kung pao chicken (light on the peanuts), beef and broccoli dishes, shrimp and snow peas, garlic chicken, Mongolian beef steak, or dishes that have meat and a vegetable. Ask for the chef to go easy on the oil.

Thai

Any of the satay dishes (chicken, shrimp, beef, or tofu), any protein or vegetable stir-fry, steamed fish, chicken or beef lettuce rolls. Avoid fatty coconut milk curries, noodles, and rice.

American

Hamburgers (without bread or on a whole-grain bun), turkey dogs, meat chili, veggie soups, kosher turkey bacon, white meat turkey burgers, white meat chicken, egg whites. Eat the toppings off your pizza, but don't eat the dough.

Indian

Chicken, lamb, beef, or shrimp tikka (grilled marinated meat skewers); any of the veggie dishes such as bhagan bharta (whipped eggplant), saag paneer (spinach with cheese), aloo gobi (marinated steamed cauliflower), vegetable jalfrezi (mixed vegetables). Avoid curries, rice, and naan bread.

Sushi

Stick to sashimi. Order your favorite rolls as hand rolls with no rice. You can do this with almost any roll.

Italian

Any chicken or fish dish, beef carpaccio, any salad (always with the dressing on the side). Avoid heavy, creamy, and sugary sauces, and don't get pasta.

French

Any steak, chicken, or fish dish; any salad (always with the dressing on the side). Avoid rich, creamy, and sugary sauces, and don't get potatoes.

Breakfast

Any egg dish with egg whites if possible, low-fat cottage cheese, sugar-free yogurt with berries, turkey bacon, smoked salmon. Avoid waffles, pancakes, bagels, muffins, doughnuts, and other pastries.

Dessert

If you cannot resist, opt for the fruit plate and/or an herbal tea such as peppermint, which aids in digestion.

part 3

SWEAT

Why Exercise?

You've made it through the Self and Science sections—now it's time to get up offa that thing and sweat! Along with the internal work and the right diet, exercise is the third key to getting and staying healthy. Obviously, it will help you lose weight—we will get to that in just a minute—but exercise offers a ton of other invaluable benefits as well. Research has clearly linked coronary heart disease, diabetes, and cancer to lifestyle. Apart from aiding in weight loss, physical activity offers a positive, healthy way to release anxieties and alleviate tensions, which can help reduce your risk of many lifestyle-related diseases. Exercise also supports mental well-being: increasing physical activity actually changes your brain chemistry, which directly influences your mood and frame of mind for the better. Among other things, physical activity triggers the release of endorphins, which act on the brain as natural tranquilizers. In addition, exercise will boost your confidence. As you start working out and getting stronger, your sense of strength in other aspects of your life will naturally flourish as well. Bottom line: the more physically fit you are, the longer you will live and the better your quality of life will be.

I know what you're saying: "That all sounds great. Now tell me how to lose my behind or my gut." In weight-loss terms, fat is energy. Those of you with a high body fat percentage have a lot of stored energy; the best way to lose it is to use it, and the best way to do that is not just to decrease your energy intake through diet but also to increase your energy expenditure through exercise. If you diet without exercise, the majority of your weight loss will be from loss of muscle; this is not just unhealthy, it's also temporary, since as soon as you abandon or even stray from your diet, the weight will come right back. The only way to lose weight and keep it off long term is to *get moving*. Exercise not only helps you burn through calories, it also helps you build, strengthen, and maintain lean muscle, which keeps your body burning fat not just during your workout, but for hours afterward—this is known as "after-burn."

Okay, up until now none of this might sound so new, but here's where I take it one step further. I train all different kinds of people, but whether they're movie stars or people I train on TV, they have one thing in common across the board: they, like you, want real results *fast*. The program outlined in the chapters that follow has been developed during years of combining the best of different exercise methods and watching my clients achieve even the most extreme weight-loss goals. When it comes to exercise, I've seen it all and I know what works. If you stick with it, my program guarantees you the same results I helped my *Biggest Loser* team achieve.

So are you ready to break a sweat and start feeling great in your body? Then let's get going: the first step in your exercise education is to learn a bit about your muscles and anatomy.

13 | Basic Anatomy

In order to custom design your own fitness regimen, you must first understand which muscles to work out when and why. There are more than six hundred muscles in the human body and about six billion muscle fibers. As fascinating as this sounds, it's way beyond the scope of this book—all you need is a basic familiarity with the major muscle groups located in your hips, upper legs, lower legs, torso, lower back, abdominals, and arms. What follows is a brief, easy-to-understand physiology lesson that will familiarize you with the basic muscle groups you will be working out and how they function within the body.

HIPS

Your hip region is made up of three main muscle groups: gluteals (your buttocks), adductors, and iliopsoas.

◈ The gluteals, or buttocks, are located on the back of the hips. This is the largest and strongest muscle set in the body, and its function is hip extension, or driving the upper legs backward. Activities that require this muscle group include walking, running, jumping, and climbing.

- ◆ The adductors are the muscles located throughout the inner thigh and are used during hip adduction, which means bringing your legs together.
- ◆ The iliopsoas, or hip flexors, is a collective term for the primary muscles on the front of your hips. The main function of the iliopsoas is hip flexion, which means bringing your knees to your chest. The iliopsoas is sometimes considered to belong to the abdominal muscle group.

UPPER LEGS

The two main muscle groups of your upper legs, or thighs, are the hamstrings and quadriceps.

- ◆ The hamstrings are located on the back of your upper legs. This muscle group is responsible for knee flexion, or bringing your heels toward your buttocks, and hip extensions.
- ◆ The quadriceps are the muscles on the front of your upper thighs. The main function of the quadriceps is knee extension, or straightening your legs.

LOWER LEGS

The two major muscle groups in your lower legs are the calves and dorsi flexors.

- ◆ The calves are located on the back of your lower legs. They are involved in plantar flexion, or extending your ankles and pointing your toes.
- ◆ Dorsi flexors are located on the front of your lower legs and are primarily used for dorsi flexion, or flexing your ankles. Strengthening the lower leg muscles is crucial to safeguard against shin splints.

TORSO

The three major muscle groups in your torso are the chest, upper back, and shoulders.

- ◆ The major muscle surrounding the chest area is the pectoralis major. It is thin and fan shaped. The pectoralis minor is a thin triangular muscle positioned beneath the pectoralis major. The chest muscles are responsible for any movement that involves pulling your arms across your body—for example, throwing and pushing.
- ◆ The muscle that comprises most of the upper back is the latissimus dorsi, or "lats," which is a long, broad muscle whose primary function is to pull your arms backward and downward, as in pulling and climbing motions.
- ◆ The shoulders are comprised of eleven muscles, of which the deltoids are the most important. The deltoids are actually composed of three separate parts, or heads. The anterior deltoid is found on the front of the shoulder and is used when you raise your arm forward. The lateral deltoid is located on the side of the shoulder and is involved when lifting your arms sideways. The posterior deltoid resides on the back of the shoulder and is used to draw your arms backward. The deltoids play a vital role in throwing, pushing, carrying, and climbing.

LOWER BACK

- ◆ Your lower back contains several muscles of which the erector spinae are the most important. Their primary purpose is torso extension, or straightening up from a bent-over position. They also assist in torso lateral flexion, or bending your torso to the side, and torso rotation, or twisting.

ABDOMINALS

The three major muscles that comprise your abdominals are the rectus abdominus, obliques, and transverse abdominus.

- The rectus abdominus, otherwise known as the eight-pack, is a long, narrow muscle that extends vertically across the front of the abdomen from the lower rib cage to the pelvis. Its main function is torso flexion, which is when you pull your torso toward your lower body.
- The obliques, which are divided into external and internal, reside on both sides of the midsection. Both sets of obliques have the same two main functions: torso lateral flexion, which is bending your body and your torso in the same direction, and torso rotation, which is turning your body away from your torso. As you can see, the obliques are used in any movement in which your torso bends laterally or twists.
- The transverse abdominus is the innermost layer of your abdominal musculature. The fibers of this muscle run horizontally across the abdomen, and its primary function is abdomen constriction.

ARMS

The three main muscles in your arms are the biceps, triceps, and forearms.

- The biceps is the prominent muscle of your upper arm and is involved in elbow flexion, or bending your arms. The biceps also assist the upper back muscles in pulling and carrying.
- The triceps is a horseshoe-shaped muscle on the back of your upper arm. Its primary function is elbow extension, or straightening your arms. The triceps

assist the chest and shoulder muscles in throwing and pushing.

◆ The forearm is comprised of two muscle groups, anterior and posterior. The anterior group on the top of your forearm facilitates wrist flexion (bending your wrist) and pronation (turning your palm downward). The posterior group on the bottom of your forearm facilitates wrist extension (straightening your wrist) and supination (turning your palm upward). Since the muscles of the forearms affect the wrists, hands, and fingers, they are extremely important in pulling, carrying, climbing, and gripping.

14 | Cardio: Everything You Need to Know

For the most part, my program makes straight cardio exercise obsolete, because the kind of resistance training I will outline in the final chapters is as effective, if not more so, at raising heart levels and burning fat as any cardio routine. That said, cardio is a great way to get a workout on the days when you are giving your muscles a rest, so it's important that you get a few basics under your belt so that you know the best times of day to do it, when to do it in relation to your resistance training, what your optimum duration and intensity are, and what types of exercise are best for you.

WHEN

If you plan on doing cardio on the same day as your resistance training, it is ideal to do it after your weight routine. While it's true that a 5-minute cardio warm-up is always necessary before any resistance training, if you do prolonged cardio beforehand you will have depleted most of your available blood sugar, which you very much need for those quick bursts of energy that resistance training requires. Additionally, cardio will fatigue your muscles before you lift a single weight, and that will prevent you from maxing out your muscle's potential when training.

On the days when you are resting your muscles and doing straight cardio alone, the best time of day is absolutely any time. The most important thing is that you do it. There is a prevailing misconception that cardio is most effective first thing in the morning on an empty stomach, the theory being that you won't have eaten in 8 to 10 hours, so there will be less blood sugar available for fuel, which will force your body to draw on and burn more of its stored energy. This is absolutely untrue. Remember the whole theory of a target fat-burning zone and low-intensity exercise being a more effective method of burning fat than high-intensity exercise? This is untrue for the same reason: a calorie is a calorie no matter what. It doesn't matter if the calories are from fat or from carbs—as long as you are burning more of them than you are taking in, you will lose weight. If anything, working out on an empty stomach could make you feel weak and could inhibit your performance. My advice is to do your cardio whenever you have the energy for it, whether it's morning or evening, on an empty stomach or following a snack. All that matters is that you are putting as much into every workout as you can—do that, and you're guaranteed to get the most out of it.

DURATION

When it comes to duration, you should do a minimum of 30 minutes and a maximum of 2 hours of cardio in any single session. On the one hand, the number of calories you burn in half an hour doesn't make it worth the trip to the gym; on the other, you don't want to exercise intensely for more than 2 hours straight, as excessive activity of this kind releases stress hormones into the body, such as cortisol, which inhibit weight loss, causing your body to react by storing fat and retaining water out of self-protection.

WHAT TO DO

You go to the gym and there are rows and rows of different machines to choose from. So how do you know which kinds of cardio are best? Do you walk, row, step, or climb your way to fitness? The answer is all of these. You should do whatever you enjoy the most—just make sure you're pushing yourself and keeping your heart rate at 85 percent of your maximum while you are doing it. Sure, there are machines that are more effective than others, but if you dread and avoid certain machines, it will be harder to motivate yourself. Make sure to keep it fresh—if you've been doing the treadmill for a while, switch to the stepper for a few weeks. If you only have access to one type of cardio machine, you can change the way you use it every once in a while so that you are avoiding the workout plateau and keeping yourself challenged and motivated.

Walking/Jogging/Running

You can perform this activity on a treadmill or outdoors. The key is to mix it up and keep it challenging. Do you walk on the treadmill but never break a stroll? Forget about it! That is totally useless. To burn maximum calories, you have to get your heart rate up to the 85 percent mark mentioned earlier. There are a few different ways of doing this: you can walk on an incline, walk fast, run, or jog, depending on what you're ready for at your current fitness level. Try performing intervals by running or jogging in quarter-mile bursts. You can also work different muscles in your legs by running backward every once in a while. Obviously you can't do this everywhere. You might also try sports drills like running sideways, or karaokes, which is trying to run sideways crossing your right foot over your left foot, then your left foot over your right foot.

Stairs

You can perform this exercise on a stair-climber or step-mill. The key to getting the most out of this exercise is taking full steps. Make sure you let your bottom leg fully extend, without touching the ground, before stepping back up. Don't lean on the machine or hold on to anything. If you need to set the speed lower in order to go hands-free, do it; you're still better off moving your upper body as you step. You can also perform this exercise sideways, and alternating your right leg over your left leg, and vice versa. This type of cardio will also tone your hamstrings, glutes, and calves, which you should bear in mind if you are working those muscle groups on the same day or on a day close to your cardio workout.

Elliptical Trainer

This machine is great because it tends to have a lot of variables built in; many of these machines have adjustable incline ramps, allowing you to work different muscles in your legs. Some also have movable handles that allow you to work your upper as well as your lower body. Obviously, if the machine you're using has these options for maximizing your session by working the upper body, use them. This machine is also good for people with knee problems, as it is low impact and easy on your joints. With elliptical trainers, it is important to increase the resistance on the machine; otherwise, gravity will be doing all the work for you. You can vary the ramp incline in order to target different leg muscles: if the ramp is inclined and you are pedaling forward, you are working the back leg muscles: the hamstrings, glutes, and calves; if the ramp is at a lower incline and you pedal backward, you are training the front leg muscles: the quads and dorsi flexors.

Swimming

Generally, swimming is kinder to your body than land-based exercise because your natural buoyancy in water helps you avoid the jarring knocks that can cause injuries. In water, you weigh about a tenth of your normal weight, and the range of motion for the less-fit person is much wider because the water supports the weight of the limbs. So swimming is a good choice for people who want to exercise, but who might have problems with weight-bearing, land-based activities. Swimming might suit those who have arthritis or back problems, weight problems, or are pregnant. To mix things and target different muscles, do vary your strokes during your swim between breaststroke, freestyle, butterfly, and backstroke.

Recumbent Bike

This form of cardio exercise is great for beginners. It is not the greatest calorie burner because your body is sitting during the exercise, so you are only working your leg muscles. Having said that, you can still pick up that resistance and push yourself as much as possible. You might want to consider doing some light arms while you bike, like biceps curls or shoulder presses, in order to get your heart rate up.

Rowing

I love this form of cardio for a change of pace. It allows you to work multiple different muscles simultaneously. You can tone your back, biceps, and quads, all while working your cardio pulmonary system as well. In order to get the most out of this exercise, keep the resistance at a minimum of 3. Make sure to press through your heels as you extend your legs. Keep your abs tight and relax your neck and shoulders. In order to target different back muscles, alternate an overhand grip with an underhand one every 5 minutes.

Jump Rope and Jumping Jacks

This is an excellent form of cardio that you can perform anywhere. No matter where you are or what the weather, you can always jump. It will take you a little time to build up an endurance for this form of cardio, so try it in intervals at first: jump one minute, rest the next, and so on. This is an outstanding form of cardio in terms of calorie burning and toning quads, hamstrings, and calves. Try different types of jumps to spot target different leg muscles. If you're jumping rope, try butt kicks or bringing your knees up as high as you can in between jumps. Try jumping on one foot at a time or alternate feet. The possibilities are endless with this simple activity.

Classes

The advantage to exercise classes is that they're a whole lot more fun than sweating it out by yourself. They also provide company for your misery, which can be a great motivator. Whether it's spinning, step, boot camp, or any other cardiovascular class, make sure it involves a minimum of 45 minutes of activity and keeps your heart rate up.

There are a lot of machines and even more ways to get a cardio workout. The ones that are best for you are, quite simply, the ones you like. Remember, this is a permanent lifestyle revolution, and you've got to find a fitness program that you can live with, even enjoy. If you honestly can't find a single activity that doesn't fill you with dread, stick to the machines or exercises that work the most muscle groups, as this will speed the metabolism, give you faster results, and help keep you motivated to stick with it.

15

Designing a Workout Routine That Works for You

These last few chapters lay out the core exercise element of my total wellness plan. Cardio is an important part of any fitness regimen. It allows for a lot of variety in terms of burning calories, and a working knowledge of the cardio fundamentals is invaluable. But if you go back to the analogy of a car being in drive, it's the next few chapters that'll kick you into turbo.

You have a basic knowledge of the major muscle groups and how they function; it's time to put that knowledge to use in designing an exercise program that's right for your unique physical attributes and fitness goals.

When it comes to working out and resistance training, there are two kinds of people: there's the skinny person who wants to get big and muscular, and there's the person who wants to shed fat and get toned. If you're in the first category, you can put this book down right now. My exercise methodologies are not going to help you gain mass. The information you will find in these pages is designed to help you develop and tone muscle, and get rid of excess fat and flab.

What is uniquely effective about my exercise program is that it does away with the traditional methods of straight cardio workout and separate weight training and instead combines the two most result-oriented types of fat burning workouts: high-intensity training and circuit training. Intensity training is when the muscles are trained aggressively to the point of fatigue, and circuit training is when a series of exercises is performed back to back with little or no recovery time in between. What makes my combo-training methods so successful is the fact that your heart rate will be elevated the entire time you are doing your strength training so that you are *burning calories* and *toning muscle simultaneously*—what this means is that basically you are going from one high-intensity set of exercises to another with as little rest in between as possible. Working out this way, you will quickly turn your body into a hyperefficient fat-burning machine not just for the duration of the workout but—and this is one of the major benefits—even after you have stopped. In the long term, this is the most effective way to lose weight and keep it off.

DURATION AND FREQUENCY

One of the first questions my new clients will ask is how long their workouts should be. My answer will vary from person to person. One of the most important elements to consider when designing a fitness regimen is practicality: you will be incorporating regular exercise into your daily schedule, so it is crucial that you don't overshoot and then get frustrated when you can't follow through.

You may have heard the U.S. Surgeon General's recommendation of 30 minutes of physical activity a day—this is intended for people who want to maintain the most basic level of fitness but not for people who want to lose weight. Honestly, the few calories you burn from daily 20–30-minute workouts over weeks are almost not worth the time it takes to go to the gym. In a week, this only works out to an expenditure of about 1,000 calories, which is fine if you are looking to maintain your current weight. But if you want to lose, you're going to have to be prepared for a bit more work.

I much prefer to use the World Health Organization's recommendation of 60 minutes at a time as a starting point for my clients—an hour being an ideal amount of time to really get the most out of your workout. Sure, this requires a little more time, but my program is guaranteed to pay off with serious results—fast. Your 60-minute workout sessions should always include a warm-up cardio session, 50 minutes of main exercise, whatever you're doing, and a cool-down session.

Every workout should start with a 5-minute warm-up cardio session. This reduces your chance of injury by literally warming up your muscles, tendons, ligaments, and joints. You should not stretch your muscles out until after you have warmed them up. The next 50 minutes of your workout is the part that will make you sweat, and make the pounds melt away.

You will be performing at levels that push you to the max in one burst of energy after another, and thus you burn calories and tone at the same time. You'll get the specifics in the exercise index and the twelve-week sample routine that follow in the next chapter.

Finally, every workout session should end with a 5-minute cool-down so that you can bring your heart rate back to normal and get blood circulating freely again without undue cardiac stress. This part of the workout should also involve stretching to help relax muscles and increase flexibility.

Apart from duration, it's also important to know how often you should be working out. In my experience, the ideal workout frequency for effecting real, lasting transformation is 5 times a week. Anything over that is unnecessary and can even be counterproductive. It is important to give your muscles a chance to rest and recover. If you are good to your body, it will be good to you.

SEQUENCE

Equally as important as duration and frequency of your workouts is which muscles you concentrate on and when. Here's the deal: it is never a good idea to work any single muscle group more than twice a week. It is much better for your muscles if you rotate the groups you work on from one day to the next. I will use the word *split* to refer to the way you divide your muscle groups across several workouts; while you are working one set of muscles, you are allowing others to recover and rebuild. Take a look at the split routine below, which divides the muscle groups into those of your body's front and those of the back. It is what I have found to be most effective in terms of preventing fatigue and over-training, and achieving maximum calorie-burning results.

MONDAY	Chest; Shoulders; Triceps; Quads; Rectus abdominus; Transverse abs
TUESDAY	Back; Biceps; Glutes; Hamstrings; Obliques
WEDNESDAY	OFF
THURSDAY	Chest; Shoulders; Triceps; Quads; Rectus abdominus; Transverse abs
FRIDAY	Back; Biceps; Glutes; Hamstrings; Obliques
SATURDAY	1 hour of straight cardio—this gives your muscles the rest and recovery time they need.
SUNDAY	OFF

This split routine might look confusing at first, but let me explain the logic. It is most advantageous to work muscle groups that have similar functions together. For example, the chest, shoulders, and triceps are all used in basic pushing and pressing motions; when you do a push-up, you are primarily working your chest muscle, but you are also working your shoulder and triceps muscles. Hence the chest–shoulders–triceps all in one day. The same goes for back and biceps muscles, whose main function is pulling; when you do a pull-up, your body is primarily using the biceps, but it also recruits the upper back muscles to complete the movement. Splitting the muscle groups and working them together by function enhances coordination and gets your muscles working together more efficiently.

Additionally, if you split your muscle groups by function, it is easy to ensure that each muscle group gets time off. In the table above, see how each muscle group gets at least 2 days off before it is worked again? This prevents overtraining by providing your muscles the time they need to repair and develop.

Now for your leg muscles: working your lower body is the most effective way to elevate your heart rate and therefore to burn more calories. For this reason, we want to work the lower body during each resistance training session. I like to divide the lower body muscles into front and back: work the front on your chest day and the back on your back day. This type of routine allows you to work your upper body and lower body in swift procession in a "super set." This drives the blood back and forth between your upper and lower body, allowing you to burn up to twice as many calories than you would from working all upper or all lower body, due to something called peripheral heart action (PHA).

PHA is at the heart of my program's guarantee of results. When you get the blood moving between the upper and lower body as constantly and furiously as possible during a workout, you greatly reduce the formation and buildup of lactic acid, which is the cause of muscle fatigue. PHA not only contributes in the short term by helping you burn more calories during your workout, it also benefits you in the long term by optimizing muscle development and preventing muscle damage or burnout.

Last of all, it is crucial to know the best sequence for performing your exercises so that you do not fatigue your muscles out of a great workout. To prevent undue fatigue, you always want to train the muscles from largest to smallest.

Here's the logic: When you exercise one of the big muscle groups, say the chest, you also recruit the smaller muscles nearby, like the triceps, in a secondary or helper capacity. Your triceps will not work as hard during a chest press as they will in a triceps curl, but if you exhaust your triceps before you even get to your chest, they'll be weak. As a result, you will not be able to give your chest the best workout possible. So if you get the big ones out of the way before you spotlight the smaller ones, your performance will improve, and this means more fat-burning lean muscle in less time.

INTENSITY

Intensity is the last piece of the puzzle. How hard should you work yourself? When it comes to weight management, there is often debate about the level of cardio intensity that is most effective for shedding weight. Some experts will say high intensity is best for losing weight; others swear low-intensity activity is more effective. Let's look at the facts.

During physical training, your body has three possible sources of energy: carbs, fat, and protein. Protein is a last resort—of the three energy sources, your body is most reluctant to draw on your protein stores. But whether your body takes energy from its carbs or its fat depends on the intensity of your workout. Training at a high level of intensity forces your body to draw on carb calories for energy—they are a more efficient source of energy, so your body goes for its premium fuel if you're working hard. If you are training at a low level of intensity, your body doesn't need to be as efficient, and it will draw on a higher percentage of fat calories for fuel.

So it sounds like low-intensity training would be more effective when it comes to losing fat, right? *Wrong.* These physiological facts have indeed led to the mistaken belief that low-intensity activity is better than high-intensity activity when it comes to burning fat and losing weight. Furthermore, this misconception has spawned the notion that people should only train within their fat-burning zones. The thing is, even though a greater percentage of fat calories is used during low-intensity exercise, the total number of fat calories used is greater during high-intensity exercise because more overall calories are burned. For example, in a half hour of low-intensity exercise, you might burn 100 calories. Of those 100 calories burned, roughly 80 percent will be fat calories, meaning you've burned 80 fat calories. In a half hour of high-intensity exercise, you might burn 300 calories. Of those 300 calories, roughly 33 percent will be fat calories, meaning you've burned 100 fat calories. Get it? Even though the percentage of fat calories burned is higher during a low-intensity workout, you're burning so many more total calories during a high-intensity workout that, percentages aside, you are still burning more fat calories with high-intensity exercise, not to mention the 200 carb calories you're burning as well. High-intensity workouts also trigger higher postworkout metabolism rates and fat afterburn.

Having said all of this, it is also true that carb calories become fat calories after a while anyway, so when it comes down to it, a calorie is a calorie is a calorie. Forget the notion of a fat-burning zone. There is only one moral of the story: burn as many damn calories as possible whenever you work out.

The one time I do strongly recommend low-intensity exercise over high is at the beginning of any fitness regimen, when you might be inclined to jump right in and give it all you've got, only to end up burning out or injuring yourself.

For the first 2 weeks of training, I make all my new clients pass the talk test during their sessions; you have to be able to carry on a conversation comfortably throughout the workout, or you're working too hard.

Once you have been exercising for several weeks, it is safe to increase your intensity, and I recommend working at about 85 percent of your maximum heart rate. To monitor your intensity, first calculate your maximum heart rate by subtracting your age from 220 if you're a woman, or 226 if you're a man. Once you have calculated what your 85 percent rate is, you can start keeping yourself at the right intensity by taking your own pulse throughout your workout. The quickest way is to count the beats for 6 seconds and then multiply by 10. You should check in every 10 minutes or so. Sometimes during weight training your heart rate will jump above that 85 percent mark, which is fine; with weights the only thing you have to be sure of is that your heart rate doesn't drop below 75 percent of your max for the duration of the workout.

When it comes to intensity, you will learn to use your own judgment. If it feels too easy, increase intensity; if it feels too difficult or your form is compromised, decrease intensity. You will find that your abilities change as you move forward, so it is important to be able to intuit the right intensity level for you. As you keep working out and getting stronger, you will have to know when and how to increase your efforts in order to keep moving toward your goals.

DON'T GET DISCOURAGED

As we discussed in chapter 6, at some point in your weight-loss journey, you will undoubtedly encounter a disappointing drop in visible results. Just as the pounds might stop falling off as your metabolism slows down to adapt to the reduced caloric intake, so too you might find that the results you're getting at the gym might hit a wall as your body tries to adapt to a new homeostasis. If you are doing the same exercises again and again, over a period of time your body will become resistant to the benefits. Do 20 lunges after not having done them in months and you'll be sore the next day; but start doing 20 lunges every day and pretty soon you won't get sore anymore. And that's when they stop doing you any good. This can be discouraging, but it can be rectified and in some cases completely circumvented.

Make sure you have not hit a plateau due to overtraining. Take a minute to assess how your body is feeling. Are you taking proper rest days in between workouts? Do you feel exhausted all the time? Has your performance at the gym fallen off? Do your legs feel heavy and hard to move? Is your resting heart rate higher than usual? If you have answered yes to a few of these questions, it is possible you might be overdoing it on the exercise, in which case it is best to raise your caloric intake by 10 percent for a week or so and take that week off from all physical activity. Let your body fully benefit from the passive calorie after burning these results from developing lean muscle, and give yourself the time your muscles need to recover. If your workout is losing steam for other reasons though, try some of my ideas to get it back on track.

Variety is the spice of life. It's also the key to keeping your workout progressing so that you are always getting the most out of it, keeping yourself challenged constantly so that you can continue to marvel at your results. It's also good just to make things interesting; if you don't mix things up every once in a while, your routine will become monotonous, unchallenging, and totally unproductive.

Switch things around at least every 4 to 6 weeks—my personal recommendation is to switch every two weeks, but the length of your program is up to you. Change your routine around the following three variables: weight load, sets/repetitions, and modality, or type of exercise. The rest of this chapter details exactly how you can change these three elements of your routine from time to time and avoid stalling on the road to fitness.

WEIGHT LOAD

The most obvious element to change in your routine is the level of resistance. No matter what piece of equipment you're using, even if it's your own body, there are many ways of decreasing and increasing the resistance level of your exercise. This can often be done in conjunction with varying your number of sets and repetitions as well. For example, for your first 6 weeks, your routine might include a set of lunges for 20 reps using just your body weight as resistance. To change this a little, you could try making it 2 sets for 10 reps, with a 15-pound dumbbell in each hand for added resistance.

SETS/REPETITIONS

Varying the number of reps and sets will constantly surprise the body, which is another way to keep your workout moving forward. For instance, you might start out with 3 sets of chest presses for 10 reps in your first program, so for a change you could do 1 set for 30 reps instead.

Apart from changing the number of sets and reps per exercise, you can also change the way you perform the rep. During a weight-lifting exercise, your muscle contracts in three distinctly different ways: (1) When you lift the weight, your muscles contract positively, or concentrically. (2) At the midpoint of the exercise when you stop moving the weight but you're still holding it, your muscles contract statically, or isometrically. (3) When you lower the weight, your muscles contract negatively, or eccentrically. You can adjust the way you do your reps by shifting focus among the three forms of muscle contraction, which means there are three ways to do almost anything in the weight room and endless ways to switch around your routine to keep it fresh and motivating.

MODALITY

Another means of varying your routine is to alternate between different exercises that work the same muscles. For example, if your routine includes the seated row machine, which works the midback, biceps, and forearms, alternate it with another machine or activity that works the same muscles and provides a change of position and pace from the seated row. Besides providing variety, alternating your exercises also trains your muscles through different ranges of motion, allowing you to target your muscles with greater accuracy.

You can refer to the exercise index for exercises listed by muscle group so that you have plenty of options from which to pick and choose to keep your program challenging, fun, and as effective as possible. You are learning this stuff so that you can take the reins—be honest with yourself about what your body is getting out of your workouts. You won't make progress unless you are constantly challenging yourself; as long as you continue to demand new things from your muscles, you will continue to see the results in your improving physique.

16 | Exercise Index

This chapter describes the safest and most productive exercises for each of the main muscle groups; they will constitute, in various combinations, the backbone of your workouts. Each description includes identification of the muscles involved, starting position, performance description, training tips, and progressions and variations for the exercise. This is your one-stop reference for all things exercise, and together with the sample 12-week program that follows, it will help you construct your own ideal workout.

Glutes and Legs

FORWARD LUNGE

Muscles targeted: glutes, quads, hamstrings, calves

Starting position: Stand with your feet hip-width apart, with your weight on your heels. Pull your abdominals in and stand with your shoulders squarely over your hips.

Performance description: Lift your left leg, leading with your heel, and step forward in an elongated stride. As your foot touches the floor, bend both knees until your left thigh is parallel to the floor and your right thigh is perpendicular to it. Your right heel will be off the floor. Exhale and press off the ball of your foot, stepping back into the starting position, and repeat, alternating legs.

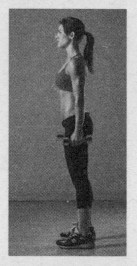
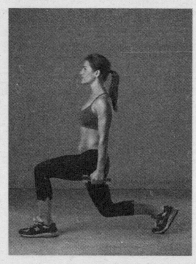

Tips: Make sure that your front knee is never allowed to travel past your toes. Keep your eyes focused forward; if you look down, you might lose balance. Keep your spine straight through the entire movement, with your shoulders always positioned squarely over your hips.

Variations
STATIC LUNGE
(beginner)
Start with your right leg a stride's length in front of the left. Bend both knees, and lower your body so that your left knee is a few inches from the ground and the right thigh is parallel to the floor. Hold in this position for a beat, then exhale, raise back up to the start position, and repeat. Complete a full set, then switch legs and repeat.

BACKWARD LUNGE
(intermediate)
Start by standing up straight with your feet hip-width apart. Step your right leg back about a stride's length behind you, and bend both knees until your left thigh is parallel to the floor and your right thigh is perpendicular to it. Hold for a beat, exhale, then press off your left foot and bring your right leg back to the starting position next to the left, and repeat, alternating legs. You will feel this version of the lunge more in your hamstrings.

PENDULUM LUNGE
(intermediate)
Stand up straight with your feet hip-width apart. Take a big step back with your left leg, bending your right knee so that your right thigh is parallel to the floor (keeping your right knee behind your toes) and your left thigh is perpendicular

to the floor. Exhale, and pressing with your right foot, swing your left leg back up and in front of you into a forward lunge so that your left thigh is parallel to the floor and your right thigh is perpendicular. Continue for a full left-leg set, then switch legs and repeat. This dynamic move gives you excellent quad definition and chiseled glutes, plus you're using more core strength to stabilize you throughout the movement.

Variations
SIDE LUNGE
(intermediate)
Stand up straight with your feet hip-width apart. Step your right leg out to the side about a stride's length, keeping it in line your left foot. Lean onto your left leg, bending at the hip, until your right thigh is nearly parallel to the floor. Using the left leg, exhale and push yourself back into starting position. Repeat the same motion with the left leg. This version of the lunge places greater emphasis on the side of your glutes and outer quads.

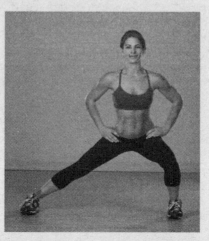

Variations
CROSS-OVER LUNGE
(advanced)

Stand up straight with your feet hip-width apart. Step your left foot diagonally forward and across the right foot. If you were standing in the middle of a clock facing the number 12, you would bring your left foot across the body and place it on the 1. Slowly lower your right knee until the left leg is parallel to the floor. Then using the left leg, exhale and push yourself back into starting position. Repeat the same motion with the right leg, only this time bring your right leg forward and place it on the number 11. This type of modified lunge places greater emphasis on the sides of your glutes.

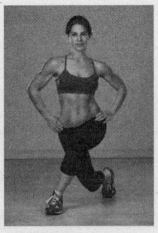

JUMPING LUNGE
(highly advanced)

Start by dropping down into a lunge position with your right leg forward and your left leg back. Exhale and jump upward, launching both legs off the floor and switching them in midair. You should land with your left foot forward and right leg back. Drop back down into a lunge and repeat. This modification is for advanced athletes only. It is to develop explosive power and core strength.

SQUATS

Muscles targeted: glutes, quads, hamstrings

Starting position: Stand with your feet apart as wide as your hips, with your weight on your heels. Keep your abs tight and stand with your shoulders squarely over your hips.

Performance description: Sit back and down as if you were to sit down onto a bench. Keep your back straight, being careful not to lean forward, and lower yourself down until your thighs are parallel with the floor. As you exhale, straighten your legs, stand back up, and repeat.

Tips: Keep your eyes focused forward. Don't lean forward or let your heels come off the ground. Don't let your knees travel forward over your toes or bow inward as you lower or

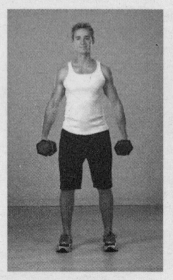 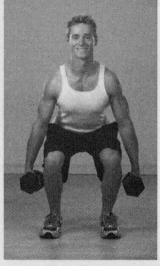

stand. Keep your belly button sucked in toward your spine as you stand back up, being careful not to arch your back.

Variations
WALL SQUAT
(beginner)
Stand about 1½ feet away from the wall in your starting position. Now slowly lower yourself down until your thighs are parallel with the ground or until you legs form a 90-degree angle. Hold this position for as long as you can, then stand back up. This exercise helps you build strength in your quads and develop your form to prepare you for performing a full squat. Don't be fooled though—this move can become advanced quickly depending on how long you hold the position and if you add any resistance to the move by holding weights or sitting on one leg only.

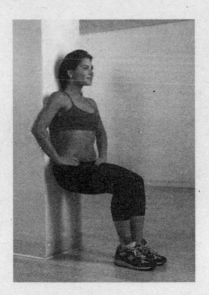

Variations
HACK SQUAT
(intermediate)

For this variation, you need one of those large bouncy balls you see at the gym known as body balls. Using a body ball can be a convenient way of keeping your home workout varied and effective. Standing with your back to the wall, place the body ball between your back and the wall and lean against the ball so that it is supporting your lower back. Now slowly lower your body until your thighs are parallel with the ground. Hold for a beat, exhale, and press back up to your starting position and repeat. This hack squat places a much greater emphasis on the quads than the glutes.

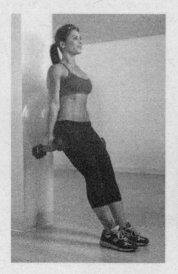
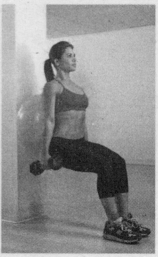

Variations
SUMO SQUAT
(intermediate)

Place your feet apart as wide as you can while also pointing toes outward. Lower your body until your thighs are parallel to the floor. Hold for a beat, exhale, press back up to starting position, and repeat. Keep your shoulders directly over your hips at all times. Don't lean forward or let your knees come out over your toes. Keep your abs drawn in and don't arch your back. This squat modification places a greater emphasis on the inner and outer thighs.

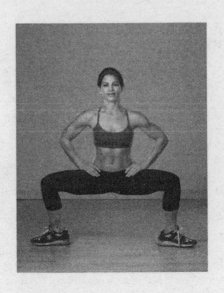

Variations

JUMPING SQUAT

(advanced)

Stand with your feet hip-width apart. Lower yourself down until your quads are parallel to the ground, abs are tight, and shoulders are over the hips, just like a regular squat. Then from the midpoint position, exhale and explode upward, jumping as high as you can. Land back down in a firm stance, reset quickly, and repeat. Jump squats utilize fast twitch muscle fibers to produce and develop speed and power. They get your heart rate way up, so they burn lots of calories, and the high resistance of jumping from the squat position gives you maximum definition in your quads and glutes.

KING SQUAT

(advanced)

This move is named after Ian King, who was the first person to perform this technique. Place a bench about 2 feet behind you. Bring your right leg up behind you and bend at the knee. Then place your right foot top down so it rests on the bench, with the edge of the bench hitting you just at the ankle. Your left leg should be planted out a little ways in front of you with toes pointing to the front. Now, bend your left leg until your left thigh is parallel with the floor. Your right knee should drop down and back toward the bench, but should never touch the ground. Keep your front left knee from going over the toe and keep your shoulders aligned over your hips. Hold for a beat and exhale, pressing back up to the starting position. Complete a full set with your left foot forward, then switch legs and repeat. The king squat develops core strength to maintain balance as well as to improve flexibility and overall leg strength.

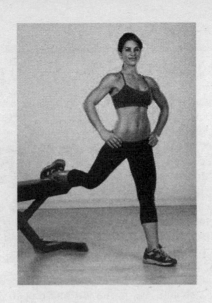

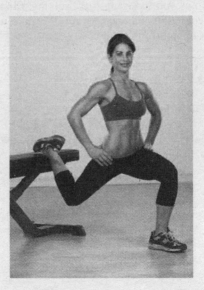

Variations
ONE-LEG SQUAT
(highly advanced)

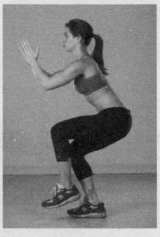

Stand on your right leg. Lift your left foot a couple inches off the ground. The same basic moves of the squat still apply. Keep your head up, don't lean forward, abs stay tight, and the right heel is on the ground. Don't let the knee go over the toe. Slowly lower yourself down as far as you can comfortably go. Exhale and stand up straight, balanced on the right leg. Continue for a full set on the right leg and then switch over to the left and repeat. This modification allows you to strengthen each leg. Since this move requires tremendous balance, you will utilize more of your core and your stabilizing muscles.

LEG PRESS

Muscles targeted: quads, glutes

Starting position: Sit down in the leg press and place your feet on the platform about shoulder width apart, toes pointed slightly out.

Performance description: Slowly lower the weight to a point where your legs are at about a 90-degree angle and your quads are just barely touching your stomach. From this point, exhale and press the weight with your quads back up to starting position, and repeat.

Tips: Always push the weight through your heels, not your toes. Never lock out your knees as you raise the weight; always keep them "soft" or slightly bent.

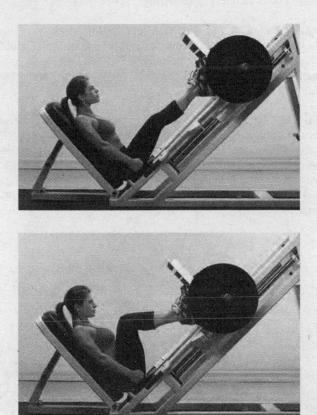

STIFF LEG DEAD LIFT

Muscles targeted: glutes, hamstrings, lower back

Starting position: Stand with your feet slightly narrower than shoulder width apart with knees slightly bent or "soft." Hold a barbell in both hands or dumbbells in each hand with your palms facing your legs. Keep your back straight and your shoulders pulled back.

Performance description: Allow the torso to slowly bend forward and the bar to lower toward the floor. Keep your knees slightly bent and your back flat throughout the entire movement. Lower the bar until your torso is almost parallel to the ground. From this position, focus on your hamstrings and exhale while slowly lifting your body and the weights back into starting position. Repeat.

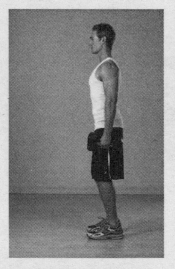 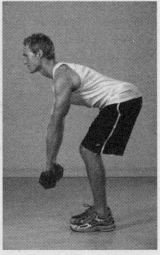

Tips: Keep your eyes focused forward to keep your back in the appropriate position. Don't round your shoulders or bend your knees too much. Be careful not to use too much weight. If done incorrectly, you can injure your lower back.

Variations
PLATFORM STIFF LEG DEAD LIFT
(advanced)

Perform a dead lift while standing on a step or low platform. If you have enough flexibility, you will be able to lower the bar beyond the level of your feet to the floor. This adds intensity to the exercise by increasing the range of motion and prolonging muscle contraction.

SEATED HAMSTRING CURL

Muscles targeted: hamstrings

Starting position: Sit on the seated curl with your back against padded back support. Place the back of your lower leg on top of the padded lever just above your heel. Secure the lap pad against your thighs just above your knees. Grasp the handles on the lap support.

Performance description: Exhale and slowly pull the weighted leg pad backward toward your hamstrings. Hold for a beat, then slowly raise the bar back to the starting position.

Tips: This exercise allows you to isolate the hamstrings better by making it difficult to cheat and engage your lower back.

Variations
LYING HAMSTRING CURL
(intermediate)

Set the ankle pads so that when you lie down on your stomach, the pads are resting just above your heels. Lie facedown on your stomach and grab the handles under the bench for stability. Make sure that the bench ends just above your knees and that your knees are just off the bench. Exhaling, curl your legs up, and bring the ankle pads as close to your hamstrings for a full contraction of the muscle. Hold the contraction for a beat, then slowly lower the weight back to the starting position and repeat. Keep your hips pressed against the machine and be careful not to lift your hips off the bench as you raise the weight.

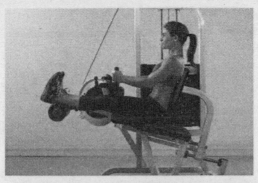

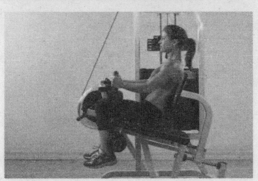

STEP UP

Muscles targeted: glutes, hamstrings, quads

Starting position: Stand facing a bench or platform with your feet hip-width apart. Place your left foot up on the step, making sure your whole foot, including the heel, is firmly placed.

Performance description: Exhale and press off your left leg to bring your right foot up onto the bench. You should have both feet firmly planted on the bench at the midpoint of this exercise. Then slowly lower your left leg back down to the ground, leaving your right foot firmly on the bench, and repeat.

Tips: Pay attention to good posture. Keep your abs drawn in and don't arch or round your back when stepping up onto the bench. Control your descent; don't let momentum drop your body when you are stepping off the bench.

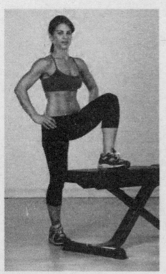
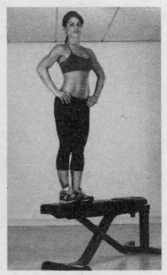

Variations
PELVIC THRUST

Muscles targeted: glutes, hamstrings

Starting position: Lie on your back in front of a bench or platform with your knees bent and your heels on the bench. Your legs should form a 90-degree angle with your knees directly above your hips, and your arms should rest on the floor at your side.

Performance description: Exhale and press your heels down into the bench, lifting your hips off the floor as high as you can. Squeeze your glutes as tight as you can for a beat, then lower back down to the floor and repeat.

Tips: Your upper arms, shoulders, and neck should remain on the floor throughout the exercise.

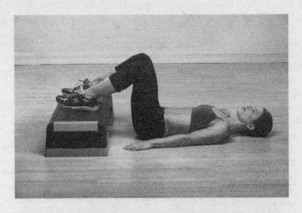

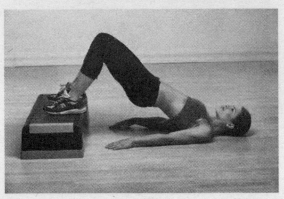

Variations
ONE-LEG PELVIC THRUST
(advanced)

Lie on your back in front of a bench or platform with your knees bent and your heels on the bench. Your legs should form a 90-degree angle with your knees directly above your hips, and your arms should rest on the floor at your side. Keeping your knees together, exhale and extend your right leg up toward the ceiling. Now, exhale and press your left heel into the bench. Lift your hips, pressing your right leg

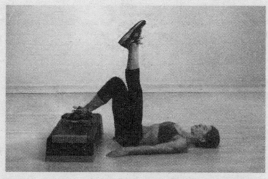

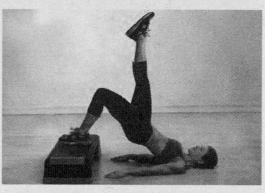

straight up toward the ceiling. Inhale and slowly lower your body back down to the floor, and repeat on the other side.

LEG EXTENSION

Muscles targeted: quads

Starting position: Set the machine so that your back is pressed firmly against the back rest. (The shin pad and back rest should be adjustable.) The seat pad of the machine should be about an inch from the back of your knees and the shin pad should be positioned just above your ankles. Sit down, bend your knees, and slide your legs under the shin pad.

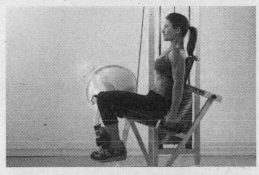

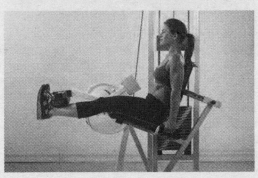

Hold on to the hands attached to the seat pad, sit up tall, and draw your belly button inward toward your spine.

Performance description: Exhale and straighten your legs to lift the ankle bar until your knees are straight. Hold this position for a beat in order to get a full contraction on the quads. Then slowly lower the weight 90 percent of the way back down and repeat.

Tips: Make sure you take the time to adjust the machine to fit your body. Don't arch your back to help you lift the weight. Don't let the ankle pad go all the way down to starting position in between reps—this motion puts too much stress on the knees.

Variations
SINGLE LEG EXTENSION
(beginner to intermediate)
You perform this exercise in the exact same way as the regular leg extension, only with one leg at a time. This allows for each leg to work individually without the stronger leg compensating for the weaker one.

BALL SQUEEZE
(intermediate)
You perform this exercise in the same exact way as a regular leg extension, only you place a medicine ball between your knees. (These are small, heavy balls, ranging in weight from 2 to 12 pounds. You will find them in most gyms, and they are excellent for adding resistance and increasing the intensity of any exercise.) As you extend your legs and lift the weight, concentrate on squeezing the ball so that it does not slip out of place. This modification incorporates more inner thigh or adductor strength into the exercise.

Back

Exercises for the upper body can be configured to spotlight different muscle groups by changing the grip that you use. Refer to this grip key as you go through the upper body exercises and their variations.

GRIP KEY

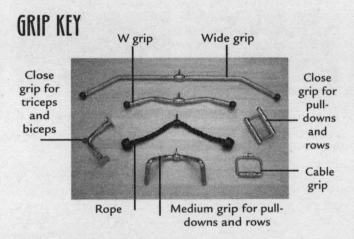

W grip   Wide grip

Close grip for triceps and biceps

Close grip for pull-downs and rows

Cable grip

Rope   Medium grip for pull-downs and rows

WIDE-GRIP LATERAL PULL-DOWN

Muscles targeted: latissimus dorsi, teres major (muscles along the side of your upper back)

Starting position: Sit down at a lat pull station and grab the bar slightly wider than shoulder width apart with an overhand grip. Place your legs under the knee pad for support.

Performance description: With your eyes forward and your

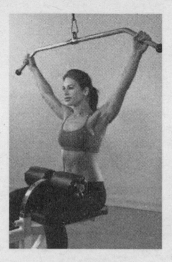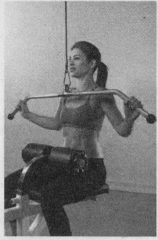

back straight, exhale and slowly pull the bar down toward your collarbone. Slowly raise your hands back above your head to the starting position and repeat.

Tips: Always keep your shoulder blades adducted (pulled inward toward your spine) during the entire movement. Do not pull the bar behind your neck. This places too much stress on your rotator cuff and can result in injury. Do not lean back or arch your back when performing the move. Leaning or arching your back engages the lower back muscles instead of the upper back muscles.

Variations

MEDIUM UNDERHAND OR REVERSE-GRIP PULL-DOWN
(beginner)

Sit down at a lat pull station and grab the bar with a reverse or underhand grip (palms facing you) with your hands shoulder width apart. Place your legs under the knee pad for support. Sit up tall and look straight ahead. Exhale and slowly pull the bar down toward your collarbone. Hold for a beat, then slowly raise the bar back up to the starting position and repeat. Don't lean back. Keep your shoulder blades adducted toward your spine throughout the entire movement. The medium grip pull-down places more emphasis on your middle upper back and your biceps.

CLOSE-GRIP PULL-DOWN
(beginner)

Sit down at a lat pull station. This time switch the bars on the lat pull-down to a close grip bar. Place your legs under the knee pad for support. Sit up tall and look straight ahead. Exhale and slowly pull the bar down toward your collarbone. Hold for a beat, then slowly raise the bar back up to the starting position and repeat. Don't lean back. Keep your shoulder blades adducted toward your spine throughout the entire movement. The close grip places more emphasis on the rhomboids, traps (upper middle back), and biceps as well as the lats.

STANDING STRAIGHT ARM LAT PULL

Muscles targeted: lattisimus dorsi and teres major

Starting position: Stand in front of a lat pull-down station. With your arms outstretched, grab the bar just wider than shoulder width apart with palms facing down. Hold the bar at your eye level.

Performance description: Keeping your elbows slightly bent and your wrists locked, exhale and pull the lat bar down toward your body in an arching motion until it touches or comes close to your thighs. Hold for a beat and inhale slowly allowing the bar to come back up to the starting position.

Tips: Make sure not to arch your back, and keep your abs tight. Don't let the lat bar raise above eye level or you'll release the contraction on your lats. Keep your wrists locked with your palms angled down toward the floor to avoid straining.

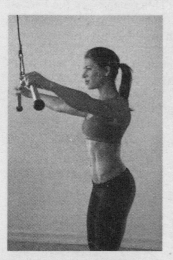 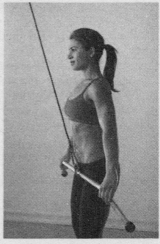

Variations
TERRY PULLS
(beginner to intermediate)

Stand in between a cable cross station with two pulleys (one in each hand). Keep one foot forward and one foot behind you. Drop on to your back knee. Your arms should be outstretched with your palms facing up. Exhale and slowly pull your elbows down to your rib cage. Hold for a beat, inhale, and then slowly release your arms back to starting position. Repeat.

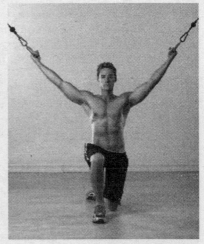

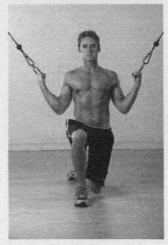

DUMBBELL ROW

Muscles targeted: upper and middle back, biceps, rear delts

Starting position: Stand straight with a dumbbell in one hand. Bend forward at the waist until your torso is almost parallel with the floor—you can brace yourself against a workout bench for support. Your knees should be bent. Your arm should be hanging down with your palm facing your thigh.

Performance description: Keeping your arm close to your torso, exhale and pull the dumbbell up until it touches the side of your chest. Hold for a beat, slowly lower the weight back down toward the floor, and repeat on the other side, with your other arm.

Tips: Keep your shoulder blades pulled in toward your spine throughout the entire exercise. Keep your elbows in next to your body and focus on pulling your elbows straight up toward the ceiling. Keep your back as straight and flat as possible, even though you are bent at waist. Focus on lifting the weight with your back muscles, not your arms.

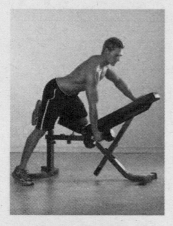
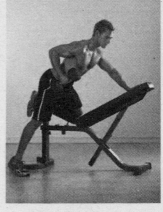

SEATED CABLE ROW

(beginner)

Sit facing the weight tower with your legs slightly bent and hip-width apart. Your feet should be placed firmly on the foot pads. Palms inward, grab the grip attached to the cable and straighten your arms out in front of you. Sit up tall, pulling your abs in, shoulders back, and the chest out. Exhale and pull the grip toward your chest, squeezing your shoulder blades together as you pull. Without leaning forward or releasing your shoulder blades, straighten your arms back to the starting position and repeat. This version of the row utilizes less of your core muscles than the dumbbell row. It is also more versatile than the dumbbell row. Like the lat

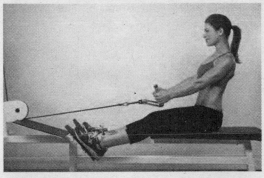

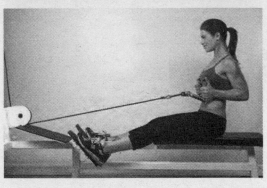

pull-down, you can change the grip bar on the row cable to vary the muscles your target in your back: You can do a wide grip row (upper and outer back muscles). You can do a close or medium grip row (midback muscles).

Variations
LOW ROW
(advanced)

Sit as you would for a seated cable row. Face the weight tower and bend your legs slightly, hip-width apart. With feet placed firmly on the foot pad, grasp the grip with your palms facing up, shoulder-width apart. Exhale and slowly pull the grip down to your stomach. This version of the seated row is great for the lower back.

SUPERMAN

Muscles targeted: lower back, glutes, hamstrings

Starting position: Lie on your stomach with your forehead on the floor and your arms straight out in front of you.

Performance description: Exhale and simultaneously lift both arms and legs a couple of inches off the floor. Hold for a beat, then lower your limbs back down to the floor and repeat.

Tips: Exhale as your raise your body up and inhale as you lower. Don't lift higher than a few inches off the ground. Keep your spine straight and your eyes focused on the floor. Don't look up because it will strain your neck.

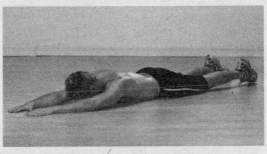

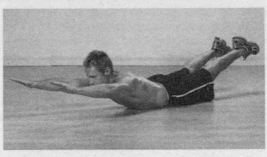

Variations

SEQUENTIAL SUPERMAN
(beginner)

Start in the same position as superman. In this version you can lessen the strain on your lower back if you are a beginner by lifting your upper body, then your lower body separately. Another option is to lift your right leg and your left arm, then your left leg and your right arm.

BACK EXTENSION

Muscles targeted: lower back, glutes, hamstrings

Starting position: Stand in the middle of the hyperextension station. Facing toward the large flat pad, lean forward until your upper thighs are placed on the pad with your hip bones just above the pad. With your legs straight, place the backs of your ankles (just above the heels) under the smaller pad. If you are a beginner, place your arms across your chest. For the more advanced version, place your hands behind your head with your thumbs behind your ears. This adds extra resistance to the exercise.

Performance description: When in position, inhale and slowly lower your upper body at the waist until it is almost perpendicular to the floor. Then exhale and slowly lift your upper body back to the starting position. Hold for a beat and repeat. For advanced exercisers, hold a weight plate against your chest to increase the resistance.

Tips: Be careful not to raise your torso beyond the point where your spine is straight and your back is flat. Control the movement and do not swing your body to cheat the exercise.

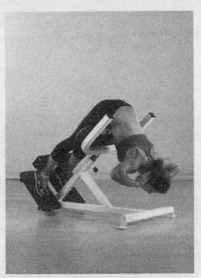

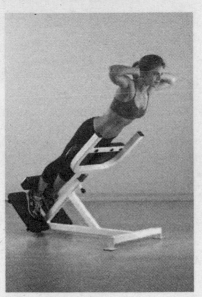

Chest

PUSH-UP

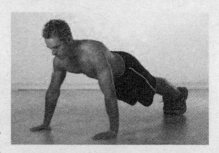

Muscles targeted: chest, shoulders, triceps, abs

Starting position: Lie face down with your legs straight out behind you and your feet together. Bend your elbows and place your palms on the floor out to the sides of your chest. Position your palms so that they are directly under your elbows. When your

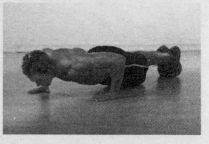

arms are bent, they should form a 90-degree angle. Your neck should be straight and your eyes should be focused on the floor in front of you. Keep your abs tight. Straighten your arms so that your body is hovering over the floor, balancing on your palms and the balls of your feet.

Performance description: Bend your elbows and lower your entire body at once until your upper arms are parallel with the floor. Exhaling, push back up to the starting position and repeat.

Tips: Keep your back straight and your eyes focused on the floor in front of you.

Variations
MODIFIED PUSH-UP
(beginner)

Find a stable elevated bench upon which to perform this exercise. If you are at home, the back of your couch or coffee table will suffice. If you are at the gym, use a weight bench. Place your palms on the bench of your choice several inches wider than shoulder width apart. Step your feet back behind you so that you are balancing in a prone position over the bench. You should be supporting your weight on the underside of your toes and the palms of your hands. Bend your elbows and lower your entire body down into push-up position. Your chest should line up with your hand position on the bench and your arms should both be in 90-degree angles at the midpoint of this exercise. Your neck should be straight and your eyes should be focused on the floor in front of you. Keep your abs tight. Exhaling, push back up to your starting position and repeat. Try to avoid doing "girl" push-ups on your hands and knees. This version is much better because it still forces you to use your core muscles, whereas the "girl" version does not.

PLYO PUSH-UP
(advanced)

Start in a push-up position hovering above the floor. Slowly lower yourself into a push-up. With an explosive burst, exhale 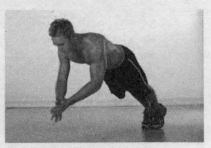 and push yourself up, lifting your hands off the floor and clapping them together. Land back in a push-up position and repeat. The plyometric push-up builds muscle by adding resistance to the regular push-up.

Variations
CLOSE-GRIP PUSH-UP
(advanced)

Start in a push-up position except keep your hands directly under your shoulders instead of outside your chest. Your legs should be straight out behind you with feet slightly apart so you are balancing on your palms and the balls of your feet. Keep your elbows pressed firmly against your torso as you slowly lower yourself down into a push-up. Exhale, press back up to the starting position, and repeat. This close-grip push-up places more emphasis on your anterior shoulders and triceps as well as your chest.

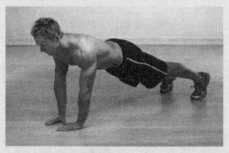

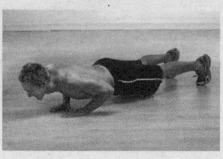

DUMBBELL CHEST PRESS

Muscles targeted: chest, shoulders

Starting position: Lie on your back on a workout bench with your feet up on the bench. (You can also perform this exercise lying on a body ball with your feet placed firmly on the floor.) Hold the dumbbells over your chest with your arms extended toward the ceiling and both palms facing forward.

Performance description: Inhale as you bend your elbows and lower the dumbbells to just above chest level. At the midpoint of this exercise, your upper arms should be parallel to the ground with your forearms perpendicular to the floor, and your knuckles should be pointed toward the ceiling. Hold for a beat, then exhale and press the weights back up to the starting position, and repeat.

Tips: Lower the weights slowly. Do not lower the weights below the edges of your outer chest or you risk straining your biceps tendon. Most people make the common mis-

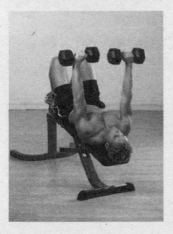
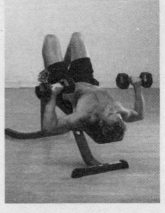

take of raising the weights above their head. Make sure to keep the weights directly over the center of your chest.

Variations
INCLINE DUMBBELL PRESS
(Intermediate)

Sit on the edge of a workout bench inclined at a 45-degree angle. Pick up your dumbbells in each hand and place them on your thighs. Position them one at a time at the base of your shoulders with your palms facing forward. Slowly lean back and get yourself firmly situated on the bench. Exhale and press the weights up to a point directly over your chest. Then inhale deeply as you lower the weights, bringing your arms to a 90-degree angle, and repeat. This variation of the dumbbell press places emphasis on the shoulders as well as the chest. Make sure not to set the bench at too steep an angle or you will place all the emphasis on your shoulders and very little on your chest.

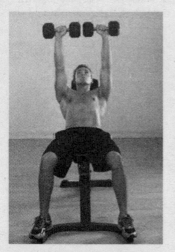 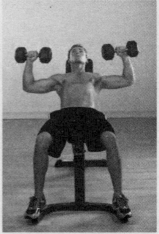

CABLE CHEST FLYS

Muscles Targeted: chest, shoulders, triceps

Starting position: Stand in between a cable cross station with two pulleys (one in each hand). Keep one foot forward and one foot behind you. Your hands should be slightly above shoulder level, with your arms open and elbows slightly bent.

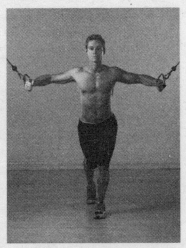

Performance Description: Exhale and slowly contract your chest, keeping arms slightly bent, and bring your hands together to meet in the center. Inhale and open your arms back to starting position and repeat.

Tips: Be sure to maintain a slight bend in your elbow throughout the entire exercise to keep the tension on your chest instead of your joints. Do not allow more than a slight bend though, or the moves become more like a press than a fly.

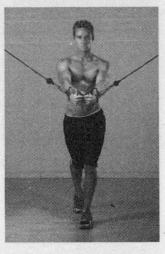

Variations
DUMBBELL CHEST FLYS
(beginner)

Lie on your back on a workout bench with your feet up on the bench. (You can also perform this exercise lying on a body ball with your feet placed firmly on the floor.) Hold the dumbbells over your chest with your arms extended toward the ceiling and both palms facing each other. Inhale, open your chest, and slowly lower the weights in a semicircle arc out to the sides of your chest. Do not lower your arms farther than parallel with the floor or you risk straining your biceps tendon. Exhale and raise the weight, again in an arc, back up to the starting position, and repeat.

INCLINE DUMBBELL FLYS
(intermediate)

Sit on the edge of a workout bench that is inclined at a 45-degree angle. Pick up your dumbbells in each hand and place them on your thighs. Raise the dumbbells over your chest with your arms extended toward the ceiling and both palms facing each other. Inhale, open your chest, and slowly lower the weights in a semicircle arc out to the sides of your chest. Do not lower your arms farther than parallel with the floor or you risk straining your biceps tendon. Exhale and raise the weight, again in an arc, back up to the starting position, and repeat. This version of the dumbbell chest fly allows you to target different muscle fibers in your chest than the flat bench press, allowing for some variety in your chest routine.

Shoulders

MILITARY SHOULDER PRESS

Muscles targeted: shoulders

Starting position: Sit on the edge of a bench or body ball with your feet flat on the floor. Hold a dumbbell in each hand and rest them on your thighs. Sit up tall with your abs drawn in, your back straight, and your eyes focused forward. Raise the weights to ear level with your palms facing forward. Your arms should be in a 90-degree angle, elbows out to the sides, forearms perpendicular to the floor, and upper arms parallel with the floor.

Performance description: Exhale and press the dumbbells up and in so that they barely touch over your head. Hold for a

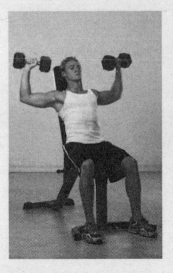 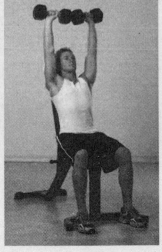

beat, inhaling, slowly lower the weights back to the starting position, and repeat.

Tips: Do not let the weights stray back and forth. Be careful not to arch your back when you raise the weights. Do not lower the weights below your ears or you'll release the contraction on your shoulders.

Variations
W SHOULDER PRESS
(intermediate)

Sit on the edge of a bench or body ball with your feet flat on the floor. Hold a dumbbell in each hand and rest them on your thighs. Sit up tall with your abs drawn in, your back straight, and your eyes focused forward. Raise the weights to ear level with your palms inward toward your ears. Your arms should be in a 90-degree angle, elbows out to the

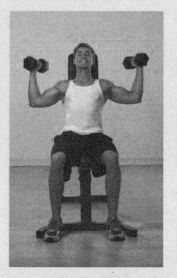
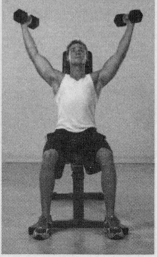

sides, forearms perpendicular to the floor, and upper arms, parallel with the floor. Exhale and extend your arms up and out as though you are trying to form the letter W with your arms. Hold for a beat. Inhale, slowly lowering the weights back to the starting position, and repeat. This shoulder press variation does work your entire shoulder, but it specifically targets the lateral head of the muscle.

REVERSE-GRIP SHOULDER PRESS
(intermediate)

Sit on the edge of a bench or body ball with your feet flat on the floor. Hold a dumbbell in each hand and rest them on your thighs. Sit up tall with your abs drawn in, your back straight, and your eyes focused forward. Raise the weights to ear level with your palms inward toward your eyes. Your arms should be in a 90-degree angle with your elbows together in front of your body. Your forearms should still be perpendicular to the floor and your upper arms parallel with the floor. Exhale and extend your arms straight up toward the ceiling. Keep your arms together throughout the entire exercise. Hold for a beat. Inhale, slowly lowering the weights back to the starting position, and repeat. This shoulder press variation does work your entire shoulder, but it specifically targets the anterior or front head of the muscle.

LATERAL SHOULDER RAISE

Muscles targeted: lateral head of the shoulder

Starting position: Stand upright with your feet shoulder-width apart and your arms at your sides. Hold a dumbbell in each hand with your palms turned toward your body.

Performance description: Keeping your arms straight, exhale and lift the weights out and up to the sides until they are parallel to the ground. Hold for a beat. Inhaling, slowly lower your arms back to the starting position, and repeat.

Tips: Keep your palms turned down toward the floor throughout the entire exercise so that you isolate the shoulders and do not engage the biceps. Do not swing the weight, lean forward, or arch your back.

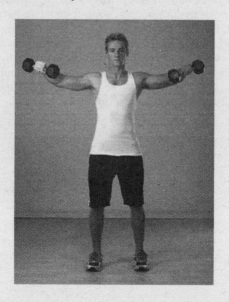

Variations
ANTERIOR SHOULDER RAISE
(beginner)

Stand upright with your feet shoulder-width apart and your arms at your sides. Hold a dumbbell in each hand with your palms facing behind you. Keeping your arms straight, exhale and lift the weights up straight in front of your torso until they are parallel to the ground. Hold for a beat. Inhaling, slowly lower your arms back to the starting position, and repeat. The anterior shoulder raise targets the front head of your shoulders.

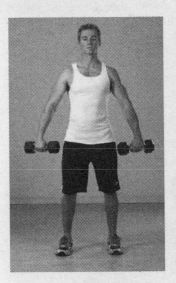
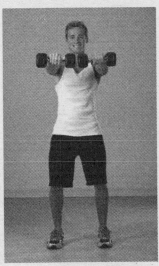

Variations
BENT-OVER SHOULDER RAISE
(beginner)

Sit on the edge of a workout bench with a dumbbell in each hand and your feet shoulder-width apart, bending forward at the waist so that your upper body is parallel with the floor. Let your arms hang straight down under your chest with your palms facing behind you. Exhale and raise the dumbbells, pulling your arms apart, up and out, until they are parallel with the floor. Hold for a beat. Inhaling, slowly lower your arms back to the starting position, and repeat. Keep a slight bend in your elbows throughout the entire movement. Be careful not to lift your torso when your raise the weight. The bent-over shoulder raise targets your rear shoulders where your back muscles and shoulders come together.

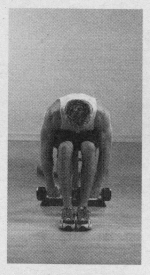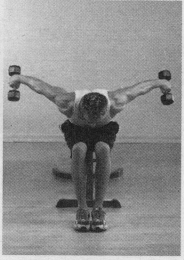

Biceps

DUMBBELL BICEPS CURLS

Muscles targeted: biceps

Starting position: Stand upright with your feet shoulder-width apart and your arms at your sides. Hold a dumbbell in each hand with your palms facing toward the sides of your body.

Performance description: Exhale, and keeping your elbows locked firmly against your rib cage, curl both arms three-quarters of the way up toward your shoulders rotating your wrist so your palm faces upward. Hold or a beat, focusing on squeezing your biceps. Inhale and slowly lower your arms back to the starting position, and repeat.

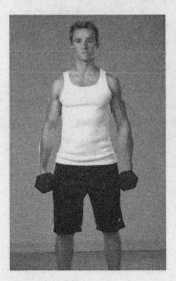 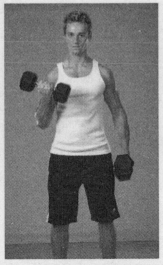

Tips: Stand straight and be careful to use slow, controlled movements. Be careful not to swing the weights. Do not lift your elbows when you raise the weights or you will engage your shoulders instead of isolating your biceps.

Variations
HAMMER CURLS
(beginner)

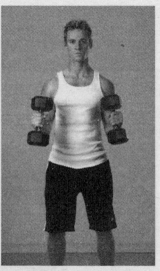

Stand upright with your feet shoulder-width apart and your arms at your sides. Hold a dumbbell in each hand with your palms facing inward toward the sides of your body. Exhale, and keeping your elbows locked firmly against your rib cage, curl both arms three-quarters of the way up toward your shoulders. Hold for a beat, focusing on squeezing your biceps. Inhale and slowly lower your arms back to the starting position, and repeat. This version of the biceps curl puts more emphasis on the forearms, as well as some muscles that reside underneath the biceps.

Variations

ZOTTMAN CURLS
(beginner)
Stand upright with your feet shoulder-width apart and your arms at your sides. Hold a dumbbell in each hand with your palms facing inward toward the sides of your body. Exhale, and as your curl your arms upward, rotate your palms in toward your body, and bring your arms up and across to the opposite shoulder. Keep your elbows locked firmly against your rib cage throughout the entire exercise and only curl both arms three-quarters of the way up toward your shoulders. Hold for a beat, focusing on squeezing your biceps. Inhale and slowly lower your arms back to starting position, and repeat. This version of the biceps curl puts more emphasis on the forearms and the inside of the biceps.

REVERSE-GRIP CURLS
(intermediate)
Stand upright with your feet shoulder-width apart and your arms at your sides. Hold a dumbbell in each hand with your palms facing behind you. Exhale, and keeping your elbows locked firmly against your rib cage, curl both arms three-quarters of the way up toward your shoulders. Hold for a beat, focusing on squeezing your biceps. Inhale and slowly lower your arms back to starting position, and repeat. This version of the biceps curl puts more emphasis on the forearms and wrists as well as the biceps.

Variations
CONCENTRATION CURLS
(intermediate)

Hold a dumbbell in your right hand and sit on the edge of a bench or a chair with your feet a few inches wider than your hips. Lean forward from your hips and place your right elbow against the inside of your right thigh, just behind your knee. The weight should hang down near the inside of your ankle. Place your left palm on top of your left thigh. Exhale and bend your right arm, curling the dumbbell three-quarters of the way up toward your shoulder. Hold for a beat,

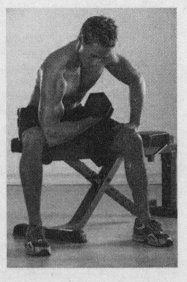

then inhale slowly, lowering the weight, and repeat. The concentration curl really isolates the biceps by taking any assistance from the back and shoulders totally out of the equation. Be careful not to cheat by leaning back for help when you are lifting the weight.

INCLINE DUMBBELL CURLS

(advanced)

Grab a pair of dumbbells in each hand and sit on a workout bench inclined at 45 degrees with your feet firmly planted on the floor. Let your arms fall at your sides with your palms facing forward. Exhale, and keeping your elbows locked firmly against your rib cage, curl both arms three-quarters of the way up toward your shoulders. Hold for a beat, focusing on squeezing your biceps. Inhale and slowly lower your arms back to the starting position, and repeat. This modification of a basic biceps curl stretches the muscle while strengthening it.

HANGING CURLS

(intermediate)

Grab a pair of dumbbells in each hand and lie facedown on a slightly inclined workout bench. Place your knees firmly on the seat part of the bench with your feet together. Let your arms fall straight down toward the floor at your sides with your palms facing forward. Exhale and curl both arms three-quarters of the way up toward your shoulders, keeping your upper arms perpendicular to the floor throughout the entire exercise. Hold for a beat, focusing on squeezing your biceps. Inhale and slowly lower your arms back to the starting position, and repeat. This modification also completely isolates the biceps by taking any assistance from the back and shoulders totally out of the equation.

Variations
CABLE CURLS
(advanced)

Stand in between a cable cross station with two pulleys (one in each hand) and feet hip-width apart. Your hands should be reaching up toward the pulleys with your palms facing up. Exhale and slowly contract your biceps curling your fists inward toward your ears. At the midpoint of this exercise, your elbows should be pointing up and out toward the pulleys. Hold for a beat, exhale, and slowly release your arms back to starting position. Repeat.

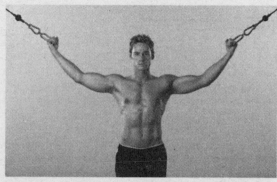

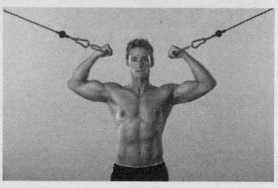

Triceps

BENCH DIPS

Muscles targeted: triceps

Starting position: Stand with your back to a sturdy bench or chair. Bend your legs and place your palms on the front edge of the bench. Position your feet in front of you so that most of your body weight is resting on your arms.

Performance description: Keeping your elbows tucked along your sides, bend your arms and slowly lower your body until your upper arms are parallel with the floor. Your hips should drop straight down toward the ground. Hold for a beat, then exhale and straighten your arms back up to the starting position, and repeat.

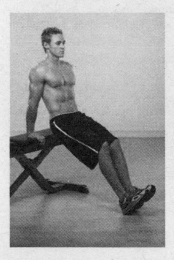 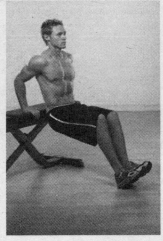

Tips: Be careful not to lower your body too far or you will overstress your shoulders. Do not lean forward or away from the bench, which also creates stress on your shoulders.

Variations
STRAIGHT LEG BENCH DIPS
(intermediate)

Start out as you would for a regular bench dip, with your back to a sturdy bench or chair. Keeping your legs straight, place your palms on the front edge of the bench or chair. You should be supporting most of your body weight with your arms. With your elbows tucked in at the side, bend your arms and slowly lower your body until your upper arms are parallel with the floor. Your hips should drop straight toward the ground. Hold for a beat, then exhale and straighten your arms so you are back to starting position, and repeat. As a variation, you can also rest your feet on a body ball. By resting your legs on the body ball, you're incorporating more of your core muscles to help you stabilize your body throughout the exercise. For a real challenge you can place one foot on the ball and hold the other straight out suspended in the air.

TRICEPS PRESS-DOWN

Muscles targeted: triceps

Starting position: Set the pulley of the cable at the topmost setting and attach a straight bar or U-shaped bar. Grasp the bar with your palms facing down and your hands about several inches from the center of the bar. Stand with your feet shoulder-width apart. Bend your elbows so that your forearms are slightly raised parallel to the ground.

Performance description: Exhale and push the bar straight down, keeping your elbows firmly pressed against your sides. Hold for a beat. Inhaling slowly, raise the bar back up to starting position and repeat.

Tips: Keep your abs tight, chest out, and shoulders back. Don't let your elbows wing out or lift up as you press and raise the weight. Be careful not to cheat by leaning forward and pushing the weight down with your shoulders. Do not let the bar raise higher than just above parallel to the floor or you are releasing the contraction on your triceps.

Variations
REVERSE-GRIP TRICEPS PRESS-DOWN
(beginner)
Set the pulley of the cable at the topmost setting and attach a straight bar. Grasp the bar with your palms facing up and your hands about several inches from the center of the bar. Stand with your feet shoulder-width apart. Bend your elbows so that your forearms are slightly raised parallel to the ground. Exhale and push the bar straight down, keeping your elbows firmly pressed against your sides. Hold for a beat. Inhaling slowly, raise the bar back up to the starting position, and repeat. This variation is easier than the overhand version because it allows the biceps to assist the triceps significantly.

ROPE PRESS-DOWN
(intermediate)
Set the pulley of the cable at the topmost setting and attach a rope grip. Grasp the rope with your palms facing each other and your thumbs up. Stand with your feet shoulder-width apart. Bend your elbows so that your forearms are slightly raised parallel to the ground. Exhale and pull the rope a few inches apart as you press it down. Keep your elbows firmly pressed against your sides. Hold for a beat. Inhaling slowly, raise the rope back up to the starting position, and repeat. This variation is more difficult because it changes the range of motion of this exercise. You not only have to press the weight down, but you also have to simultaneously pull it to the outside of your body.

DUMBBELL TRICEPS EXTENSION

Muscles targeted: triceps

Starting position: Hold a dumbbell in each hand and sit on a bench with your feet shoulder-width apart. Extend both arms directly over your head so that they are perpendicular to the floor and in line with your body.

Performance description: Inhaling, bend your arms slowly, lowering the dumbbells behind your head. Keep your elbows close to your head and pointed straight up throughout the entire exercise. Lower the weight until you feel a stretch in the back of your arms. Exhale and raise the weight following a slight arc back up to the starting position.

Tips: Be careful not to hit the back of your head when raising the weight. Do not let your elbows flare out so that you can maintain emphasis on the triceps, not the shoulders.

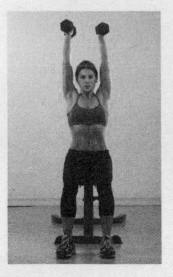
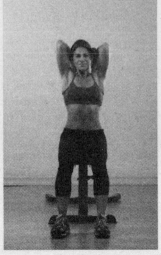

Variations
DUMBBELL FRENCH PRESS
(intermediate)

Lie on a bench with your feet placed together on top of the bench. Hold a dumbbell in each hand and straighten your arms directly over your shoulders with your palms facing each other. Pull your abdominals in and keep your head and neck relaxed on the bench. Keeping your upper arms perpendicular with the floor, inhale and bend your elbows, lowering the dumbbells back and down until they are alongside either ear. Then exhale and straighten your arms to raise the dumbbell back up to the starting position, and repeat.

TRICEPS KICK-BACKS

Muscles targeted: triceps

Starting position: Hold a dumbbell in each hand and stand with your feet hip-width apart and a slight bend in your knees. Bend over at the waist so that your torso is slightly above parallel with the floor. Bend both elbows so that your upper arms are locked at your sides parallel to the floor. Your forearms should be perpendicular to the floor.

Performance description: Keeping your upper arms still, straighten your arms behind you until the end of the dumbbell is pointing down toward the floor with your palms facing in toward your body. Hold for a beat and inhale, slowly lowering your arms back to the starting position, and repeat.

Tips: Keep your abs tight and your back flat. Do not let your upper arms move throughout the entire exercise.

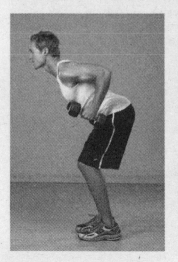 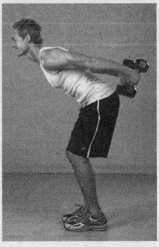

Abs

BASIC CRUNCH

Muscles targeted: rectus abdominus

Starting position: Lie on your back with your knees bent and your feet placed flat on the floor about hip-width apart. Place your hands behind your head so that your thumbs are behind your ears. Do not lace your fingers together. Keep your elbows open and out to the sides. Keep your chin up and off your chest.

Performance description: Take a deep breath, then exhale while curling up and forward until your shoulder blades are lifted off the floor. Hold for a moment at the top of the movement, fully exhale all of the air in your lungs for complete contraction of the abs, then slowly lower yourself back to the floor. Another option if you can't stop pulling on your neck is to cross your arms across your chest. Keep your tongue pressed on the roof of your mouth to help alleviate straining the back of your neck.

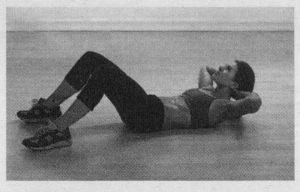

Tips: Pick a spot on the ceiling and keep your eyes focused on it to avoid pulling on your neck, and do not bring your elbows in or forward. When crunching, pull—do not push—your stomach out. Instead, pull your belly button inward toward your spine. Try to imagine you're lifting your chin up—not forward—toward the ceiling.

Variations
CRUNCH TWIST
(beginner–intermediate)
Get into the starting position of a basic crunch. Place your right hand behind your head so that your right thumb is behind your right ear. Place your left hand at your side on the floor. Crunch up and twist your torso to the left, raising your right armpit up and across the body toward your left knee. Lower back to the floor and repeat. You can switch sides or perform a full set on each side. The crunch twist still works the rectus abdominus, but it places greater emphasis on the external obliques.

Variations
OBLIQUE SIDE CRUNCH
(beginner–intermediate)

Get into the start position of a basic crunch. From there, roll your knees over to the left side and rest your legs on the floor in a bent position. Keep your torso straight. Take a deep breath and then exhale while crunching up and forward until your shoulder blades lift off the floor. Hold for a moment at the top of the movement, fully exhale for complete contraction of the abs, and then slowly lower back to the floor. Complete a full set and then repeat with legs resting to your right. The oblique side crunch still works the rectus abdominus, but it places greater emphasis on the internal obliques.

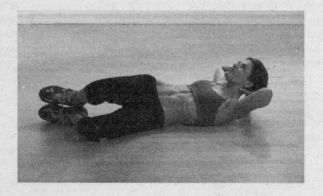

BALL CRUNCH
(intermediate)

Sit on top of the body ball with your feet placed flat on the floor about hip-width apart. All the basic crunch tips still apply: hands behind your head so that your thumbs are behind your ears, elbows out, eyes and chin up. Slowly pull your abs inward as you lean back on the ball so that your entire back from your tailbone to your shoulders is resting on the ball. Exhale as you curl up and forward until your shoulder blades come off the ball. Hold the midpoint position for a beat, then inhale, lowering slowly back down onto the ball. For a real challenge, try performing the same exercise with one foot elevated several

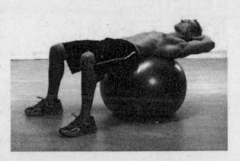

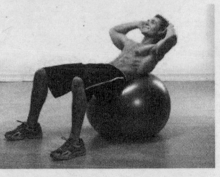

inches off the floor. Your hip stabilizer and abdominals will have to work much harder to keep you balanced throughout the movement. The ball crunch is a much more intense crunch because it allows for a fuller range of motion while performing the exercise as well as developing core stability to help you balance on the ball.

LEGS-UP CRUNCH
(intermediate)
Lift your legs off the floor and hold them up toward the ceiling, then perform a basic crunch. This modification engages the lower abs and hip flexors as well as the upper abs.

Variations
REVERSE CRUNCH
(intermediate)

Lie on your back with your feet off the floor, knees bent, and ankles together. Bring the tops of your quads inward and onto your stomach so that you don't swing your legs to gain momentum during the movement. This also helps you isolate your lower abs during the crunch instead of engaging the hip flexors. Relax your head, neck, and shoulders, resting them on the floor. Lift your pelvis off

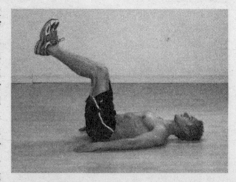

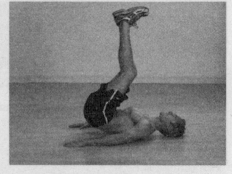

the floor and curl it toward your rib cage. Make sure to fully exhale while you're crunching in order to maximize the contraction. If you really want a challenge, hold your arms out at your sides and several inches off the floor. This helps to further isolate your abs, prohibiting your arms from assisting in the crunch by pressing off the floor with your hands. The reverse crunch specifically targets the lower abs and transverse abs.

Variations
BICYCLE CRUNCH
(intermediate)

Lie on your back with your legs up and bent at the knee, so your thighs are perpendicular to the floor and your calves are parallel to the floor. Draw your belly button in toward your spine, and press your lower back into the floor. Rest your hands behind your head with your thumbs behind your ears. Exhale as you extend your right leg out straight; simultaneously lift your shoulders off the floor, keeping your elbows open, and bring your right armpit and left knee toward each other. Inhale, then exhale as you repeat the exercise, using the opposite arm and leg. Keep the movement slow and controlled. The bicycle targets your rectus abdominus (inner and outer obliques).

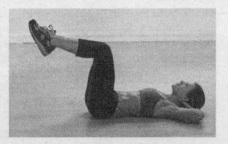

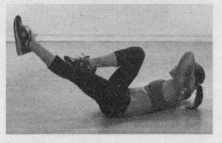

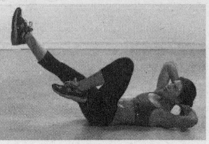

Variations
WEIGHTED CRUNCH
(advanced)

Lie on your back in the basic crunch position. Take a dumb-bell, weight plate, or medicine ball and hold it above or on top of your chest. You can also hold the weight behind your head, but it places a greater strain on your back. Now perform a basic crunch, but you will raise the weight as you raise your chest up toward the ceiling. The weighted crunch is for building a "six-pack." This modification targets your upper abs, and adding weight to the exercise stimulates muscle growth. If you still have weight to lose, I do not recommend this move. If you build your stomach muscles underneath fat, it will only create the illusion of a bigger tummy.

Variations
DOUBLE CRUNCH
(advanced)

Lie on your back in basic crunch position. Eyes and chin are up; elbows are out and open. Exhale and simultaneously crunch your upper and lower body at once (you are simply performing a basic crunch and reverse crunch at the same time). Think about touching the bottom of your rib cage and your hips together. The double crunch targets your entire rectus abdominus. It is very difficult but very effective.

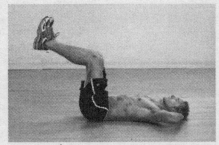

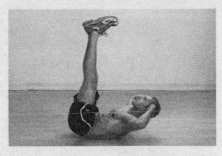

HANGING ABS

Muscles targeted: lower abs, transverse abs, hip flexors

Starting position: Slide your arms into two padded loops suspended from a bar or frame. Keep your feet together and let your legs hang down slightly in front of your body.

Performance description: Keeping your feet together, exhale while slowly raising your knees upward toward the ceiling. If you are capable, try continuing this motion, and rolling your pelvis upward toward the ceiling, touch your knees to your elbows.

Tips: Keep your head up and eyes forward. Don't swing your legs to gain momentum. Be slow, focused, and controlled.

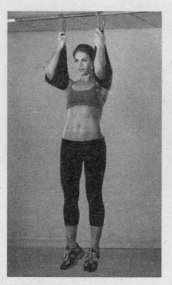 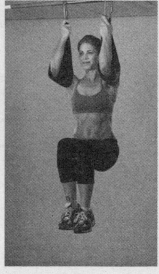

Variations
HANGING ABS WITH A TWIST

(intermediate)

Get into the hanging abs starting position. Keeping your feet together, exhale, and while slowly raising both your knees, try to pull the left knee to the right outside of your body. Slowly lower your legs back to the starting position and repeat on the opposite side. Modifying the move in this way not only works the lower and transverse abs but also targets the internal obliques.

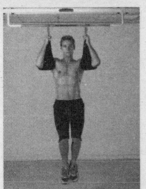
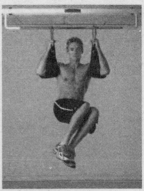

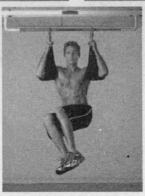

Variations
STRAIGHT LEG HANGING ABS
(advanced—highly advanced)

Get into the hanging abs starting position. Keep your legs straight while raising them up and out until they are parallel with the floor. For a challenge, try raising your legs all the way up toward the ceiling and touch the bar above your head with your feet.

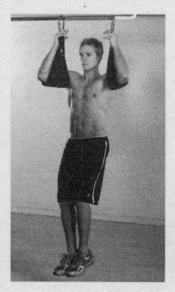
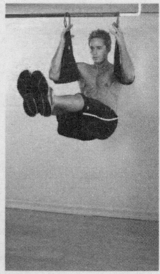

PLANK

Muscles targeted: rectus abdominus, lower back, chest, shoulders

Starting position: Start in a push-up position, except keep your hands directly under your shoulders instead of outside your chest. Legs are out straight behind you with feet together. You are balancing on your palms and the balls of your feet. Hold this position for as long as you can. Work your way up to 1 minute.

Performance description: Nothing to perform here. Just hold this static contraction as long as you can. It's a lot harder than it sounds!

Tips: Be conscious of keeping your spine neutral (straight). Keep your eyes focused on the ground in front of you. Don't arch your back. Imagine you are pulling your belly button up toward the ceiling.

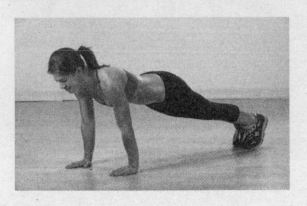

Variations
PLANK TWISTS
(intermediate)

Start in plank position. Maintaining this position, exhale and rotate your torso by bringing your right knee in toward your left armpit. Return to the starting position, then repeat with the left knee toward the right armpit. Plank twists work not only the rectus abdominus but the internal obliques as well.

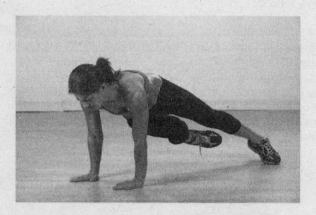

Variations
SIDE PLANK
(advanced)

Start by lying on your right side, legs extended, with your left foot stacked on top of your right. Support your body weight on your right elbow and right hip. Rest your left arm on the side of your body. Keeping your belly button pulled in, exhale and raise your hips up until your body forms a straight line from head to toe. Hold for as long as you can. Try and work

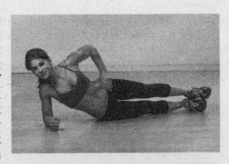

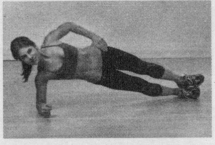

up to holding this position for a minute. To give yourself a challenge, raise your hips up until your body forms a straight line from head to toe, then slowly lower your hips back down to the starting position, and repeat. Perform a full set, then switch to the other side, and repeat. Make sure and keep your chest out, shoulders back, and spine straight. This version of the side plank targets your inner and outer obliques.

Variations
UNSTABLE PLANK
(advanced)

Start in the plank position. Keeping your belly button pulled in, exhale as you lift your left arm and reach forward, simultaneously lifting your left leg off the floor. Breathe deeply as you hold the pose for 10 seconds. Lower your limbs back to the plank position, then repeat with the opposite arm and leg. If you find this too difficult, you can work up to it by lifting only one limb at a time.

EXTENDED PLANK
(advanced)

Start in a straight plank position, except instead of placing your hands under your shoulders, bring your hands together and place them on the floor in front of you (about 3 inches in front of your head). This variation places much greater emphasis and intensity on the rectus abdominus because you are not able to utilize your arms as pillars to support your body weight.

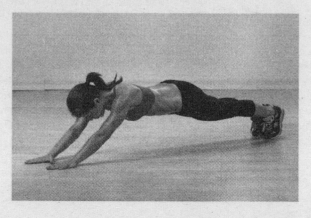

LYING LEG RAISES

Muscles targeted: lower abs, transverse abs

Starting position: Lie on your back with your legs straight out in front of you. Place your hands under your hips with your palms flat on the floor for support.

Performance description: Exhale slowly and lift your legs up without bending them until they are perpendicular with the floor. Inhale and slowly lower them back toward the floor, but do not let them touch the floor. Hold them for a beat several inches off the ground, then repeat.

Tips: Keep your legs straight the entire time. Do not lift your head or arch your back.

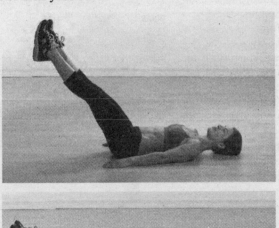

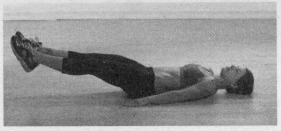

Variations

SCISSORS

(intermediate)

Lie on your back with your legs straight out in front of you. Place your hands under your hips with your palms flat on the floor for support. Raise your legs to a 45-degree angle about 1½ feet off the floor. Exhale and scissor your legs back and forth, bringing your right leg over your left and your left leg over your right. Move your legs up and down an imaginary ladder, scissoring them as high as you can and as low as you can without touching the floor. Start out scissoring for 30 seconds and try to work your way up to a minute. Scissors work lower abs as well as inner thighs.

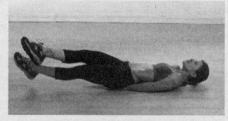

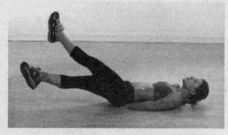

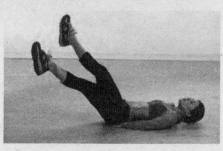

Variations
HOLLOWMAN
(intermediate–advanced)

Lie on your back with your legs straight out in front of you, arms resting at your sides. Exhale and raise your legs about 6 inches off the floor. Simultaneously crunch up with your lower body and reach your hands out toward your feet. At midpoint of this pose, you should feel as though your midsection is hollow. Hold this pose for as long as you can, trying to work your way up to a minute. Keep your eyes on the ceiling with your chin up. This modification works your entire abdominus rectus.

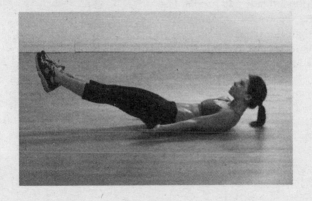

Variations
LATERAL LEG RAISES
(advanced)

Lie on your back with your legs directly above your hips perpendicular to the floor. Your arms should be straight out to your sides as if forming a T with your torso. Your palms are down on the floor for support. Inhale and slowly lower your legs directly over to your right side. Bring them as low as you can without touching the floor. Keeping your legs totally straight, exhale and raise them back up to the starting position. Switch over to the left side and repeat. Lateral leg raises predominantly target the obliques as well as the lower abs and hip flexors.

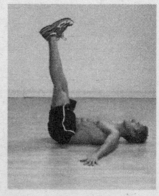

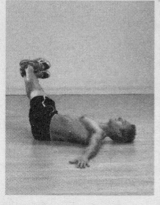
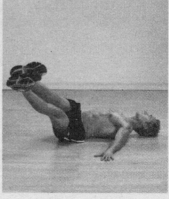

RUSSIAN TWIST

Muscles targeted: rectus abdominus, internal and external obliques, transverse abs

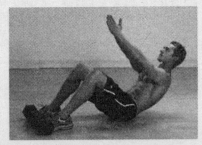

Starting position: Lie on your back with your knees bent and your feet placed flat on the floor about hip-width apart. You can place weights on your feet to help keep them rooted on the ground. Now sit about halfway up and place your hands directly out in front of you. Your arms are straight with palms together and your chin is up and off your chest.

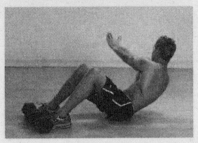

Performance description: Take a deep breath and then exhale while slowly twisting your torso as far to the right as you can manage without changing the

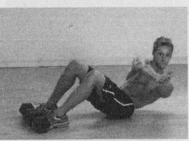

angle of your torso from the floor. Now inhale slowly and rotate your torso back to the starting position. Repeat by rotating torso to the left side.

Tips: Keep you chest out and your shoulders back; careful not to round your back. Hold for a moment at the top of the movement, fully exhale for complete contraction of your abs, and then slowly return to center or start position.

Interval Cardio Moves

MOUNTAIN CLIMBERS

Muscles targeted: cardiopulmonary system, chest, shoulders, lower abs, transverse abs

Starting position: Start in a plank (see p. 231) position with your feet hip-width apart.

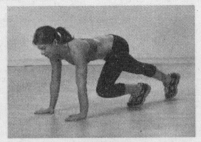

Performance description: Bend your right knee and with a springing movement, bring your right thigh under the right side of your torso. Quickly spring back out to the starting position while jumping your left knee in toward your torso. Try to work up to a minute of mountain climbers in a row.

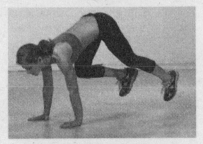

Tips: Keep your pace as fast as possible.

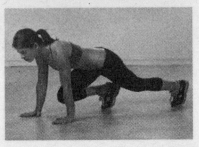

Variations
SQUAT THRUSTS
(intermediate)

Start in a plank position with your feet hip-width apart. Bend your knees and jump both feet forward simultaneously to your hands so that you're in a crouch position. Quickly extend your legs and jump both feet back behind you into the starting position, and repeat. Make sure to keep your abs tight and don't let your lower back sag or drop. Try to work up to a minute of squat thrusts in a row.

STEP PLYOS

Muscles targeted: cardiopulmonary system, quads, inner and outer thighs

Starting position: Stand facing a vertical step box or 12-inch platform with your right foot placed on top of it and your left foot on the floor behind it.

Performance description: Pushing off the right foot, hop up into the air and land with your left foot in the center of the box and your right foot on the floor. Exhale each time you push off the bench. Keep a fast pace in order to keep your heart rate up.

Tips: Make sure you push off the foot that is placed on the step, not the foot on the floor. Always land with a slightly bent knee. Keep your abs tight and your pace fast.

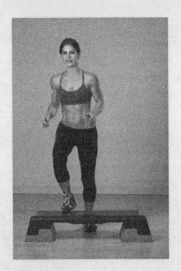

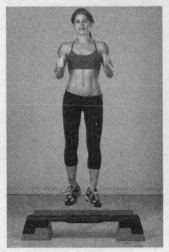

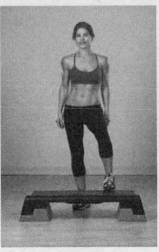

SQUATTING LATERAL STEP PLYOS

(intermediate)

Stand sideways with your right foot on the center of a vertically placed step box or 12-inch platform and your left foot on the floor. Pushing off the right foot, hop laterally up and to your right, landing with your left foot in the center of the box and your right foot on the floor. Repeat on the left leg. Exhale each time you push off the bench. Keep a fast pace in order to keep your heart rate up.

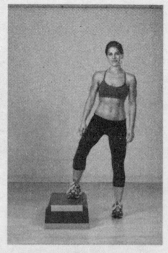

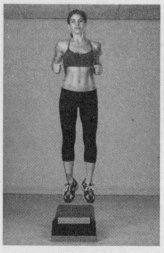

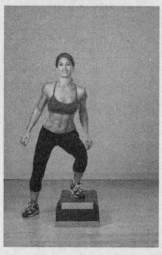

HIGH KNEES

Muscles targeted: cardiopulmonary system, abs, hips, quads, calves

Starting position: Stand with your feet hip-width apart.

Performance description: Jog in place, bringing your knees up in front as high as you can.

Tips: Keep your pace as fast as possible. Lean your upper body back and tilt your pelvis forward and upward toward the ceiling.

BUTT KICKS

Muscles targeted: cardiopulmonary system, hamstrings

Starting position: Stand with your feet hip-width apart.

Performance description: Now, jog in place, but bring your heel up to your buttocks each time you lift your foot.

Tips: Keep your pace as fast as possible and really try to kick yourself in the buttocks.

Now that you know the moves, it's time to get moving. Here's a sample 12-week workout program that I have designed to get you into the right rhythm. Use the exercises and your own experience to guide you. From now on, this is all about you. I've given you the tools, the know-how, and the challenge: now it's up to you to go out, do the work, and reap the ultimate reward.

WEEKS 1 AND 2

Perform 3 sets of 15 reps for each circuit with a comfortable amount of weight resistance that doesn't compromise your form. Try not to rest in between sets or circuits. (G = Grip, DB = Dumbbell)

Monday	Chest Shoulder Triceps Quads Rectus Abs	Circuit 1 Push-Ups Squats	Circuit 2 Dumbbell Chest Flys Sumo Squats
Tuesday	Back Biceps Hamstrings Glutes Obliques	Circuit 1 Wide-G Lat Pull Downs Stiff-Leg Dead Lifts	Circuit 2 Medium-G Seated Cable Row Static Lunges (on each leg)
Wednesday	REST	REST	REST
Thursday	Chest Shoulders Triceps Quads Rectus Abs	Circuit 1 DB Chest Presses Hack Squats	Circuit 2 DB Chest Flys Sumo Squats
Friday	Back Biceps Hamstrings Glutes Obliques	Circuit 1 Terry Pulls Side Lunges	Circuit 2 Close-G Pull-Downs Leg Press
Saturday	1 hour cardio of your choice: 5-minute warm-up at 70% of max heart rate 5-minute cool-down at 65% of max heart rate		
Sunday	REST	REST	REST

Circuit 3	Circuit 4	Circuit 5
Bench Dips	Lateral Raises	Triceps Extensions
Leg Extensions	Jumping Jacks (1 minute)	Jump Rope (1 minute)
	Basic Crunches	Scissors

Circuit 3	Circuit 4	Circuit 5
Back Extensions	Dumbbell Curls	Concentration Curls
Hamstring Curls	Jumping Jacks (1 minute)	Jump Rope (1 minute)
	Bicycle Crunches	Russian Twists

REST	REST	REST

Circuit 3	Circuit 4	Circuit 5
Bench Dips	Shoulder Press	Kick-Backs
Leg Extensions	Jumping Jacks (1 minute)	Jump Rope (1 minute)
	Basic Crunches	Reverse Crunches

Circuit 3	Circuit 4	Circuit 5
Supermans Pelvic Thrusts	Hammer Curls	Reverse Curls
	Jumping Jacks (1 minute)	Jump Rope (1 minute)
	Plank Twists	50 Bicycles

50 minutes must be at 80-85% of max heart rate

REST	REST	REST

WEEKS 3 AND 4

Perform 2 sets of 15 reps for each circuit with a comfortable amount of weight resistance that doesn't compromise your form. Try not to rest in between sets or circuits. (G = Grip, DB = Dumbbell)

Monday	Chest Shoulder Triceps Quads Rectus Abs	Circuit 1 Push-Ups Squats Mountain Climbers (1 minute)	Circuit 2 Dumbbell Chest Flys Sumo Squats Mountain Climbers (1 minute)
Tuesday	Back Biceps Hamstrings Glutes Obliques	Circuit 1 Wide-G Lat Pull-Downs Stiff-Leg Dead Lifts Butt Kicks (1 minute)	Circuit 2 Seated Cable Row Forward Lunges Butt Kicks (1 minute)
Wednesday	REST	REST	REST
Thursday	Chest Shoulders Triceps Quads Rectus Abs	Circuit 1 Dumbbell Chest Presses Hack Squats Mountain Climbers (1 minute)	Circuit 2 Dumbbell Chest Flys Sumo Squats Mountain Climbers (1 minute)

Circuit 3	Circuit 4	Circuit 5
Bench Dips	Lateral Raises	Triceps Extensions
Leg Extensions	Jumping Jacks (1 minute)	Jump Rope (1 minute)
Jumping Jacks (1 minute)	Basic Crunches	Scissors

Circuit 3	Circuit 4	Circuit 5
Back Extensions	Dumbbell Curls	Concentration Curls
Seated Hamstring Curls	Jumping Jacks (1 minute)	Jump Rope (1 minute)
Jumping Jacks (1 minute)	25 Bicycles	Russian Twists

REST	REST	REST

Circuit 3	Circuit 4	Circuit 5
Bench Dips	Military Shoulder Presses	Triceps Kick-Backs
Leg Extensions	Jumping Jacks (1 minute)	Jump Rope (1 minute)
Jumping Jacks (1 minute)	Crunches	Reverse Crunches

WEEKS 3 AND 4 (continued)

Friday	Back Biceps Hamsgrings Glutes Obliques	Circuit 1 Terry Pulls Side Lunges Butt Kicks (1 minute)	Circuit 2 Close-G Pull- Downs Leg Presses Butt Kicks (1 minute)
Saturday	1 hour cardio activity of your choice: 5-minute warm-up at 70% of max heart rate 5-minute cool-down at 65% of max heart rate		
Sunday	REST	REST	REST

Circuit 3	Circuit 4	Circuit 5
Supermans	Hammer Curls	Reverse Curls
Jumping Jacks (1 minute)	Jumping Jacks (1 minute)	Jump Rope (1 minute)
	Plank Twists	50 Bicycles

50 minutes must be at 80-85% of max heart rate

REST	REST	REST

WEEKS 5 AND 6

Perform 3 sets of 12 reps for each circuit. Build up your weight resistance as much as possible without compromising your form. Try not to rest in between sets or circuits. (G = Grip, DB = Dumbbell)

Monday	Chest Shoulder Triceps Quads Rectus Abs	Circuit 1 Push-Ups Squats Mountain Climbers (1 minute)	Circuit 2 Incline Dumbbell Flys Sumo Squats Mountain Climbers (1 minute)
Tuesday	Back Biceps Hamstrings Glutes Obliques	Circuit 1 Close Grip Rows Stiff Leg Dead Lifts Butt Kicks (1 minute)	Circuit 2 Medium-G Pull-Downs Backward Lunges Butt Kicks (1 minute)
Wednesday	REST	REST	REST
Thursday	Chest Shoulders Triceps Quads Rectus Abs	Circuit 1 Cable Cross-overs Hack Squats Mountain Climbers (1 minute)	Circuit 2 Cable Flys Sumo Squats Mountain Climbers (1 minute)

Circuit 3	Circuit 4	Circuit 5
Bench Dips	Lateral Shoulder Raises	Triceps Press-Downs
Leg Extensions	while doing Jumping	Jump Rope (1 minute)
Jumping Jacks	Jacks (1 minute)	50 Scissors
(1 minute)	20 Ball Crunches	

Circuit 3	Circuit 4	Circuit 5
Low Rows	Dumbbell Biceps Curls	Concentration Curls
Lying Hamstring	while doing Butt Kicks	Jump Rope (1 minute)
Curls	(1 minute)	50 Crunch Twists
Jumping Jacks	50 Bicycles	
(1 minute)		

REST	REST	REST
Circuit 3	Circuit 4	Circuit 5
Bench Dips	W Shoulder Presses	Triceps Kick-Backs
Leg Extensions	while doing Jumping	Jump Rope (1 minute)
Jumping Jacks	Jacks (1 minute)	25 Leg Raises
(1 minute)	Basic Crunches	

WEEKS 5 AND 6 (continued)

Friday	Back Biceps	Circuit 1	Circuit 2
	Hamstrings	Terry Pulls	Wide-G Lat
	Glutes Obliques	Cross-over	Pull-Downs
		Lunges	Leg Presses
		Butt Kicks	Butt Kicks
		(1 minute)	(1 minute)
Saturday	1 hour cardio of your choice: 5-minute warm-up at 70% of max heart rate 5-minute cool-down at 65% of max heart rate		
Sunday	REST	REST	REST

Circuit 3	Circuit 4	Circuit 5
Supermans	Hammer Curls while	Reverse Curls
One-Leg Pelvic	doing Jumping Jacks	Jump Rope (1 minute)
Thrusts	(1 minute)	50 Bicycles
Jumping Jacks	Side Plank (1 minute)	
(1 minute)		

50 minutes must be at 80-85% of max heart rate

REST	REST	REST

WEEKS 7 AND 8

Perform 3 sets (reps may vary) for each circuit. Build up your weight resistance as much as possible without compromising your form. Try not to rest in between sets or circuits. (G = Grip, DB = Dumbbell)

Monday	Chest Shoulder Triceps Quads Rectus Abs	Circuit 1 Push-Ups Squats Step Plyos (1 minute)	Circuit 2 Inclilne Dumbbell Chest Flys Sumo Squats Step Plyos (1 minute)
Tuesday	Back Biceps Hamstrings Glutes Obliques	Circuit 1 Wide-G Rows Stiff Leg Dead Lifts Butt Kicks (1½ minutes)	Circuit 2 Medium-G Pull-Downs Backward Lunges Butt Kicks (1½ minutes)
Wednesday	REST	REST	REST
Thursday	Chest Shoulders Triceps Quads Rectus Abs	Circuit 1 Cable Cross-overs Hack Squats Step Plyos (1 minute)	Circuit 2 Cable Flys Sumo Squats Plyo Steppers (1 minute)

Circuit 3	Circuit 4	Circuit 5
Bench Dips	Lateral Shoulder Raises	Triceps Press-Downs
Leg Extensions	while doing Jumping	Jump Rope (1½ minutes)
Jumping Jacks	Jacks (1½ minutes)	50 Scissors
(1½ minutes)	20 Ball Crunches	

Circuit 3	Circuit 4	Circuit 5
Low Rows	Dumbbell Biceps Curls	Concentration Curls
Hamstring Curls	while doing Butt Kicks	Jump Rope (1½ minutes)
Jumping Jacks	(1½ minutes)	50 Crunch Twists
(1½ minutes)	50 Bicycles	

REST	REST	REST
Circuit 3	Circuit 4	Circuit 5
Bench Dips	Military Shoulder Presses	Triceps Kick-Backs
Leg Extensions	while doing Jumping	Jump Rope (1½ minutes)
Jumping Jacks	Jacks (1½ minutes)	25 Leg Raises
(1½ minutes)	Basic Crunches	

Friday	Back Biceps Hamstrings Glutes Obliques	Circuit 1 Terry Pulls Crossover Lunges Butt Kicks (1½ minutes)	Circuit 2 Wide-G Lat Pull-Downs Leg Presses Butt Kicks (1½ minutes)
Saturday	1 hour cardio of your choice: 5-minute warm-up at 70% of max heart rate 5-minute cool-down at 65% of max heart rate		
Sunday	REST	REST	REST

Circuit 3	Circuit 4	Circuit 5
Supermans	Hammer Curls while	Reverse Curls
One-Leg Pelvic	doing Jumping Jacks	Jump Rope (1½ minutes)
Thrusts	(1½ minutes)	50 Bicycles
Jumping Jacks	Side Plank (1½ minutes)	
(1½ minutes)		

50 minutes must be at 80-85% of max heart rate

REST	REST	REST

WEEKS 9 AND 10

Perform 3 sets (reps vary per exercise) for each circuit. Build up your weight resistance as much as possible without compromising your form. Try not to rest in between sets or circuits. (G = Grip)

Monday	Chest Shoulder Triceps Quads Rectus Abs	Circuit 1 5 Push-Ups (hold midpoint, position for 3 sec. on each rep) Wall Squat (1 minute) Step Plyos (1 minute)	Circuit 2 15 Incline Dumbbell Flys Sumo Squats (hold midpoint position 1 minute) Step Plyos (1 minute)
Tuesday	Back Biceps Hamstrings Glutes Obliques	Circuit 1 5 Wide-G Lat Pull-Downs (hold midpoint position for 3 sec. on each rep) 20 Step-Ups Jog (1½ minutes)	Circuit 2 12 Med.-G Rows 20 Side Lunges Jog (1½ minutes)
Wednesday	REST	REST	REST

Circuit 3	Circuit 4	Circuit 5
15 Triceps Press-Downs	Anterior Shoulder Raises while doing Jumping Jacks (1½ minutes)	Triceps Extensions
5 Leg Extensions (hold midpoint position for 5 sec. on each rep)	20 Double Crunches	Jump Rope (1½ minutes)
Jump Rope (1½ minutes)		10 Hanging Abs

Circuit 3	Circuit 4	Circuit 5
20 Back Extensions	Hold Squat position and do 10 Alternating Dumbbell Biceps Curls on each arm	Cable Curls
5 Hamstring Curls (hold midpoint position for 5 sec. on each rep)	Jog (1½ minutes)	Side Planks
Jog (1½ minutes)	20 Russian Twists	Jog (1½ minutes)

REST	REST	REST

WEEKS 9 AND 10 (continued)

Thursday	Chest Shoulders Triceps Quads Rectus Abs	Circuit 1 5 Dumbbell Chest Presses (hold start position for 5 sec. on each rep) 10 One-Leg Squats Squatting Lateral Step Plyos	Circuit 2 15 Cable Flys Sumo Squats (hold midpoint position 1 minute) Squatting Lateral Step Plyos (1 minute)
Friday	Back Biceps Hamstrings Glutes Obliques	Circuit 1 5 Terry Pulls (hold start position for 5 sec. on each rep) 30 Cross-Over Lunges (1½ minutes)	Circuit 2 8 Med.-G Rows 25 fast Leg Presses Jog (1½ minutes)
Saturday	1 hour cardio of your choice: 5-minute warm-up at 70% of max heart rate 5-minute cool-down at 65% of max heart rate		
Sunday	REST	REST	REST

Circuit 3	Circuit 4	Circuit 5
15 W Shoulder Presses	12 Lateral Shoulder Raises	Triceps Kick-Backs
Leg Extensions	Mountain Climbers (1½ minutes)	Jog (1½ minutes)
Jumping Jacks (1½ minutes)	20 Double Crunches	25 Leg Raises

Circuit 3	Circuit 4	Circuit 5
20 Supermans	10 Hammer Curls	Reverse Curls
50 Pelvic Thrusts	30 Lunges	Jog (1½ minutes)
Jog (1½ minutes)	Side Planks	10 Side Leg Raises
	Jog (1½ minutes)	

50 minutes must be at 80-85% of max heart rate

REST	REST	REST

WEEKS 11 AND 12

Perform 2 sets (reps vary per exercise) for each circuit. Build up your weight resistance as much as possible without compromising your form. Try not to rest in between sets or circuits. (G= Grip)

Monday	Chest Shoulder Triceps Quads Rectus Abs	Circuit 1 25 Push-Ups 15 Jumping Squats	Circuit 2 10 (heavy) Dumbbell Chest Flys 15 Jumping Sumo Squats
Tuesday	Back Biceps Hamstrings Glutes Obliques	Circuit 1 10 Wide-G Rows 30 Step-Ups Jog (2 minutes)	Circuit 2 12 Close-G Pull-Downs 20 Side Lunges Jog (2 minutes)
Wednesday	REST	REST	REST
Thursday	Chest Shoulders Triceps Quads Rectus Abs	Circuit 1 15 Dumbbell Chest Presses (laying on ball) 15 Jumping Squats High Knees (1 minute)	Circuit 2 15 Cable Flys Sumo Squats (hold midpoint position 1 minute) Squatting Lateral Step Plyos (1 minute)

Circuit 3	Circuit 4	Circuit 5
20 Bench Dips	12 Bent-Over Shoulder	Triceps Extensions
Backward Lunges	Raises	Jog (2 minutes)
Jog (2 minutes)	Jog (2 minutes)	15 Hanging Abs
	25 Double Crunches	
	20 Ball Crunches	

Circuit 3	Circuit 4	Circuit 5
20 Back Extensions	12 Stiff Leg Dead Lifts	15 Hammer Curls
12 Lying Hamstring	with Dumbbell Biceps	100 Bicycles
Curls	Curls	Jog (2 minutes)
Jog (2 minutes)	Jog (20 minutes)	
	25 Russian Twists	

REST	REST	REST

Circuit 3	Circuit 4	Circuit 5
12 Shoulder Presses	12 Lateral Shoulder	15 Triceps Kick-Backs
Wall Squat	Raises	Jog (2 minutes)
(1 minute)	Mountain Climbers	Plank (1 minute)
Jump Rope	(1½ minutes)	
(2 minutes)	25 Double Crunches	

WEEKS 11 AND 12 (continued)

Friday	Back Biceps Hamstrings Glutes Obliques	Circuit 1 8 (Heavy) Terry Pulls 20 Jumping Lunges	Circuit 2 10 Dumbbell Rows 20 fast Leg Presses Stairs (2 minutes)
Saturday	1 hour cardio of your choice: 5-minute warm-up at 70% of max heart rate 5-minute cool-down at 65% of max heart rate		
Sunday	REST	REST	REST

Circuit 3	Circuit 4	Circuit 5
12 Low Rows	20 Hammer Curls	10 Reverse Curls
Reverse Planks (1 minute)	30 Step-Ups	Jog (2 minutes)
Jog (2 minutes)	20 Side Planks	100 Bicycles

50 minutes must be at 80-85% of max heart rate

| REST | REST | REST |

17 Keeping It Going

Okay, you're still reading, so I can only assume you're doing the work and are well on your way to achieving your weight-loss goals. Feels pretty good, right? No matter where you are on your journey, you should consider yourself on your way, and now it's time for some parting advice.

My program is about *total* health. Those changes you're implementing in your life? PERMANENT, Baby. Just because you might get into a size 8, or have a six-pack to show off for summer, doesn't mean you can throw caution to the wind, no *way*. I am hoping that after all you've read and learned here, you will now look at your life in new ways, with deeper insight and understanding. The bottom line is you can never go back to your old way of life, if you want to maintain your success. You're on the wagon, my friend. Like any recovery, just because you're rehabilitated doesn't mean you can't relapse.

All that soul-searching and honest examination from the Self section has to continue. As you grow and change, so does the need for self-discovery. It's an ongoing process, and it can continue only with the right motivation and mindset. All those behavior modifications and healthy life-affirming habits you learned have to stay in place every day for the rest of your life. I know, it sucks, it's hard, *whatever*. It's the truth, and you're better off hearing it.

Your metabolic type and your unique nutritional needs will never change. You have to stay conscious of your ideal macronutrient ratios so that your metabolism can continue to function optimally, and you will be less likely to backslide. You can't go back to eating garbage. You should still avoid those bad fats, processed grains, and refined sugars. The good news is that it will get easier as you become accustomed to the feeling of giving your body what it thrives on, and eventually it will become a gut instinct to make the right food choices.

Here's where you do catch a break: Once you have reached your ideal weight, your exercise and diet regimes can come down a notch in intensity. Since you don't need to lose weight, you don't need to create caloric deficits anymore. So go back and refigure your active metabolic rate (AMR), which will have changed since you're in better physical condition. Now that you're maintaining rather than losing, your AMR represents the number of calories you can have in a day, rather than a number you have to stay below. Obviously you should keep it healthy, but you can eat more.

You don't have to work out like a fiend anymore, either. You're not trying to burn through excess stores of fat. To maintain your weight and your strength, three or four hours a week is enough. Stick to the guidelines and principles I laid out for you in the Sweat section so that you continue to maximize your time at the gym, but you don't have to go all out anymore. The hard part's over—relax and enjoy the rewards.

Now, go with God, Baby—you *can* do this. You're doing it right now. If you get lost, go back to the beginning, I'll be right here if you need me!

Index